AF580522

S. Karger AG, P.O. Box, CH–4009 Basel (Switzerland) www.karger.com

Library of Congress Cataloging-in-Publication Data

Names: Nestlé Nutrition Workshop (95th : 2020 : Online), author. | Black, Maureen M., editor. | Singhal, Atul, editor. | Hillman, Charles H., Dr., editor. | Nestlé Nutrition Institute, issuing body.
Title: Building future health and well-being of thriving toddlers and young children / editors, Maureen M. Black, Atul Singhal, Charles H. Hillman.
Other titles: Nestlé Nutrition Institute workshop series ; v. 95. 1664-2147
Description: Basel ; Hartford : Karger ; Switzerland : Nestlé Nutrition Institute, [2020] | Series: Nestlé nutrition institute workshop series, 1664-2147 ; vol. 95 | Includes bibliographical references and index. | Summary: "This book covers the content of the 95th Nestle Nutrition Institute Workshop (held virtually in September, 2020), which explored the current scientific research, challenges, and opportunities of cementing a healthy foundation for life in toddlers and young children. The key issues presented offer valuable insights for health care providers, policy makers, and researchers on how appropriate nutrition, nurturing caregiving, and environment can influence the development and health of children up to five years of age"-- Provided by publisher.
Identifiers: LCCN 2020047731 (print) | LCCN 2020047732 (ebook) | ISBN 9783318068658 (hardcover ; alk. paper) | ISBN 9783318068665 (ebook)
Subjects: MESH: Child Nutritional Physiological Phenomena | Feeding Behavior | Child Development | Child Health | Infant Health | Congress
Classification: LCC RJ216 (print) | LCC RJ216 (ebook) | NLM W1 NE228D v.95 2021 | DDC 613.2083/2--dc23
LC record available at https://lccn.loc.gov/2020047731
LC ebook record available at https://lccn.loc.gov/2020047732

Printed on acid-free and non-aging paper (ISO 9706)
ISBN 978–3–318–06865–8
e-ISBN 978–3–318–06866–5
ISSN 1664–2147
e-ISSN 1664–2155

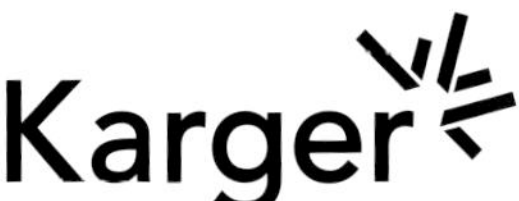

Basel · Freiburg · Hartford · Oxford · Bangkok · Dubai · Kuala Lumpur · Melbourne · Mexico City · Moscow · New Delhi · Paris · Shanghai · Tokyo

Contents

For more information on related publications, please consult the NNI website: www.nestlenutrition-institute.org

Published online: December 3, 2020

Black MM, Singhal A, Hillman CH (eds): Building Future Health and Well-Being of Thriving Toddlers and Young Children. Nestlé Nutr Inst Workshop Ser. Basel, Karger, 2020, vol 95, pp VII–IX (DOI: 10.1159/000511525)

Preface

The health and well-being of young children are not only central to their families, but also central to the United Nations Sustainable Developmental Goals and to the health and well-being of future generations. Thriving children are dependent on nutrition and physical activity: beginning with the health of parents prior to conception and continuing through the prenatal period into infancy, toddlerhood, early childhood, and across adolescence. Nutrition, which includes not only food but also eating patterns, influences the rapid physical and brain development that occurs throughout this period, establishing the foundational processes that influence health throughout life, including the origins of chronic illnesses. Likewise, physical activity early in life contributes to children's health and cognitive functions, and leads to healthy patterns of physical activity throughout life.

Children's nutrition and physical activity habits are formed at home, with influences from the broader society, including neighborhoods, child care centers, and schools. Influences also extend beyond the local setting to include the geopolitical environment, climate, and, most recently, the COVID-19 pandemic. The importance of thriving children and building healthy habits is the topic of the 95th Nestle Nutrition Institute Workshop entitled *Building Future Health and Well-Being of Thriving Toddlers and Young Children*, which was held virtually (due to COVID-19) in September 2020.

The first section of this book comprises 5 chapters that cover broad aspects of nutrition in toddlers and young children. The first chapter sets the scene and describes how behaviors such as increasing autonomy and impulsivity can make toddler mealtimes uniquely challenging. These behaviors also render the assessment of toddler diets particularly difficult, but despite limited research in this age group, it is clear that many toddlers and young children throughout the world are at risk for both under- and overnutrition: the so-called double burden of malnutrition. Using Brazil as an example, the section considers how changes in lifestyle and eating habits have led to problems of malnutrition in young children worldwide. Malnutrition during a critical developmental period, in turn, has major consequences on health throughout life, as described in the chapters reviewing the impact of poor nutrition in young children from low-, middle-, and high-income countries. In particular, the section highlights the complex causes and health consequences of obesity in preschool children, a major global public health issue. Collectively, this section emphasizes the common nutritional problems seen in young children worldwide, their consequences on short- and long-term health, and why solutions to these complex problems must involve families, schools, governments, and the food industry.

The second section of the volume includes 5 chapters that address the food and eating transition that occurs from infancy to toddlerhood and early childhood. As child care enrollment increases among infants and toddlers, child care settings are increasingly important in the development of healthy nutritional habits for young children. The section includes an illustration of the development of nutrition recommendations for children in licensed child care settings, ranging from breastfeeding infants to facilitating healthy eating patterns among toddlers. The development of taste begins with prenatal flavor experiences through the maternal diet and the emergence of the olfactory and gustatory systems, which are linked to children's subsequent acceptance of solid foods. Caregivers play important roles in introducing new food and helping their children develop food preferences and healthy eating habits as they gain expertise in self-feeding. However, toddlerhood brings increases in children's autonomy and self-regulation. Toddlers may be hesitant to try new foods or demanding regarding favorite foods. Caregivers desire information and strategies to help their children participate in family meals and develop a healthful relationship with food and eating. This section also addresses the changing nutritional needs of toddlers, with information on toddlers' micronutrient needs and the controversial role of sugar in children's diet.

The third section of the volume includes 4 chapters that focus on the influence of various health factors and lifestyle behaviors (e.g., motor skill acquisition, physical activity, and nutrition) on the developing brain from early childhood to adolescence. Each chapter is focused on a set of distinct, yet related, health factors that affect brain development (including brain structure and/or function), as observed via alterations in cognitive or behavioral outcomes. As such, this section represents a cohesive collection that provides a window into lifestyle factors that may shape health and wellness during childhood and across the lifespan. Health behaviors such as physical activity and nutritional intake are essential to optimizing brain development, which is a necessary precursor for school-based learning and achievements. Specifically, the building blocks of motor skill acquisition and provision of key nutrients are fundamental to the development of physical activity and healthy eating behaviors during childhood and adolescence, respectively, which have demonstrated benefits for brain health, cognition, and academic achievements. Given that children have become increasingly inactive and that diet quality has deteriorated in recent years, such behaviors have contributed to public health and educational concerns. By incorporating opportunities for physical activity and the provision of a high-quality diet, children are best positioned to thrive both physically and cognitively.

Maureen M. Black
Atul Singhal
Charles H. Hillman

Published online: December 3, 2020

Black MM, Singhal A, Hillman CH (eds): Building Future Health and Well-Being of Thriving Toddlers and Young Children. Nestlé Nutr Inst Workshop Ser. Basel, Karger, 2020, vol 95, pp X–XI (DOI: 10.1159/000511523)

Foreword

According to the World Health Organization, the early child period, i.e., from birth to 5 years of age, is considered the most important developmental phase throughout the lifespan.

This period of a child's life is fundamental in building the foundation for physical growth, development, health, and social and emotional skills. In fact, the first 3 years of life, which include a good portion of toddlerhood, shapes a child's brain structure in preparation for lifelong learning. The development of fine motor skills, language, and social and behavior skills are all categories that children, particularly toddlers, are seeking to master.

As it was stated in the 2018 Global Nutrition Report, although the number of children who are stunted decreased, millions of children are still affected by stunting and wasting (150.8 million [22.2%] and 50.5 million children under 5 years of age, respectively), while the number of children who are overweight is steadily rising (38.3 million children under 5 years of age). In such significant disparities, appropriate nutrition, stable, responsive, and nurturing caregiving, as well as safe and supportive environments are the 3 critical elements of healthy child development.

The 95th Nestle Nutrition Institute Workshop *Building Future Health and Well-Being in Thriving Toddlers and Young Children*, was the first NNI Workshop presented 100% virtually, and explored in some detail the current scientific research, challenges, and opportunities of cementing a healthy foundation for life in toddlers and young children.

The program brought together three outstanding experts in the areas of health care, public health, and developmental science. The first session, chaired by Prof. *Atul Singhal* (University College London), focused on the nutritional challenges in toddlers and young children across the globe, such as nutrient deficiencies as well as overweight/obesity, which can be especially detrimental during an important period of child development and growth. The theme of the second session, led by Prof. *Maureen M. Black* (RTI International and University of Maryland School of Medicine), elucidated the journey from infancy to toddlerhood and the role of nutrition in it. A large focus of the scientific debates was also given to social aspects, i.e., responsive, responsible, and nurturing caregiving.

The third session of the workshop on health behavior and the developing brain aimed to explain the steps of motor skill development and the role of physical activities and nutrition in cognitive development and learning abilities of a child. This session, chaired by Prof. *Charles H. Hillman* (Center for Cognitive and Brain Health – Northeastern University), concluded this fascinating scientific forum.

The key issues provided by this 3-day workshop offer valuable insights for health care providers, policy makers, and researchers on how appropriate nutrition, nurturing caregiving, and environment can influence the development and health of children up to 5 years of age.

We gratefully acknowledge the three Chairpersons Atul Singhal, Maureen M. Black, and Charles H. Hillman, who assembled this outstanding scientific program. We would also like to thank all speakers and experts in the audience who have contributed to the content of the workshop and scientific discussions.

Finally, we express our gratitude to Dr. Tamara Lazarini, her team in Brazil, and the Nestlé Nutrition Institute team in Switzerland for their efforts to make this workshop happen during this challenging time of a world pandemic.

Dr. Natalia Wagemans
Global Head, Nestlé Nutrition Institute
Vevey, Switzerland

Ms. Nicole E. Logan
Department of Psychology
Northeastern University
125 NI
360 Huntington Avenue
Boston, MA 02115
USA
logan.n@husky.neu.edu

Ms. Katherine M. McDonald
Department of Psychology
Northeastern University
125 NI
360 Huntington Avenue
Boston, MA 02115
USA
mcdonald.kath@husky.neu.edu

Dr. Kameron J. Moding
Department of Human Development and Family Studies
Purdue University
1200 West State Street
West Lafayette, IN 47907
USA
kmoding@purdue.edu

Dr. Elizabeth A. Offord
Nestlé Research, Vers-chez-les-Blanc
Nestlé Institute of Health Sciences
Route du Jorat 57
CH–1000 Lausanne 26
Switzerland
elizabeth.offord-cavin@rdls.nestle.com

Prof. Andrew M. Prentice
MRC Unit The Gambia
London School of Hygiene and Tropical Medicine
Atlantic Boulevard, Fajara
PO Box 273, Banjul
The Gambia
aprentice@mrc.gm

Dr. Lorrene D. Ritchie
Division of Agriculture and Natural Resources
Nutrition Policy Institute
University of California
2115 Milvia Street, Suite 301
Berkeley, CA 94704
USA
lritchie@ucanr.edu

Prof. Atul Singhal
Childhood Nutrition Research Centre
Population, Policy and Practice Research and Teaching Department
UCL Great Ormond Street Institute of Child Health
30 Guilford Street
London WC1N 1EH
UK
a.singhal@ich.ucl.ac.uk

Ms. Elyse Homel Vitale
Strategy and Operations
Child Care Food Program Roundtable
c/o Community Partners
1000 N Alameda Street, Suite 249
Los Angeles, CA 90012
USA
elyse@ccfproundtable.org

Mr. Nathaniel Willis
Division of Nutritional Sciences
University of Illinois at Urbana-Champaign
317 Louise Freer Hall
906 South Goodwin Avenue
Urbana, IL 61821
USA
nwillis3@illinois.edu

Published online: November 6, 2020

Black MM, Singhal A, Hillman CH (eds): Building Future Health and Well-Being of Thriving Toddlers and Young Children. Nestlé Nutr Inst Workshop Ser. Basel, Karger, 2020, vol 95, pp 1–11 (DOI: 10.1159/000511518)

Toddler Development and Autonomy: Baby-Led Weaning, Neophobia, and Responsive Parenting

Maureen M. Black

Department of Pediatrics, University of Maryland School of Medicine, Baltimore, MD, USA, RTI International, Research Triangle Park, NC, USA

Abstract

Toddlerhood, the period from 12 to 36 months, represents striking changes in children's development. Along with mastery of skills such as walking, talking, self-feeding, sleeping through the night, and bowel and bladder control, toddlers strive for autonomy as they learn to regulate their emotions. Toddlers' increasing autonomy impacts feeding behavior and may increase or restrict their food exposures. Baby-led weaning, allowing infants to participate in the family meal by selecting food and feeding themselves, exposes children to the family diet. Food neophobia, a normal developmental phase whereby children reject novel foods, may limit children's exposure to high-quality foods. Food preferences formed during toddler and preschool years often persist into adulthood, making toddlerhood an ideal time to help children build healthy habits. Toddlerhood can be both joyful and challenging as children acquire new skills and assert their autonomy. Effective parenting practices include providing age-appropriate structure and opportunities for toddlers, reading toddler's signals, and responding promptly, appropriately, and with nurturance. Responsive parenting ensures that toddlers receive the guidance and nurturant care needed to develop healthy feeding behavior and emotional well-being.

Introduction

Toddlerhood (age 12–36 months), the transition between infancy and the preschool years, is a period of multiple developmental changes. During toddlerhood, children consolidate many of the skills that begin to emerge during infancy. Walking with a wide-based gait becomes steady walking, running, and jumping. Single words become multiword sentences. Being fed by a caregiver becomes self-feeding along with food preferences. These advances represent toddlers' increasing neurocognitive, motor, and language skills along with their desire for autonomy and their emerging ability to regulate their behavior and emotions. This chapter begins with a review of the development changes that occur during toddlerhood and then addresses toddler eating behavior, focusing on how toddlers' advancing developmental skills impact their eating behavior, dietary preferences, and mealtime habits.

Toddler Development

The home is a central environment for toddlers [1], with caregivers helping toddlers develop daily habits and routines. Patterns developed in toddlerhood related to diet, sleep, and physical activity set the stage for lifestyle patterns throughout childhood and adolescence [2]. Toddlers' increasing autonomy impacts their feeding behavior and may increase or restrict their food exposures. Dietary patterns established during toddlerhood often persist into adulthood, making toddlerhood an ideal time to increase children's dietary diversity [1]. Toddlers benefit from parenting that is responsive, while ensuring that their introduction to the family meal includes exposure not only to nutrient-rich food but also to healthy mealtime behaviors.

Growth, Motor Skills, and Physical Activity

During toddlerhood, the rate of weight and height gain slows down from the rate of growth during infancy, body fat declines, muscle tone increases, and body proportions change as toddlers take on the physical appearance of children rather than infants. Excess weight gain during toddlerhood can increase the risk of overweight and obesity throughout childhood and adolescence [3, 4], which renders toddlerhood an ideal time to establish healthy dietary and physical activity habits. In 2014, 14.5% of US children aged 2–4 years who were participating in the Special Nutrition Supplemental Program for Women, Infants, and Children were obese (age- and sex-specific body mass index ≥ 95th percentile) [5], underscoring the increasing rates of excess weight gain in toddlers that have been observed globally.

Gross motor skills progress rapidly as toddlers become adept at walking and running without falling. Balance improves, and they are eager to jump and climb. Gradually toddlers build coordination, although skills such as riding a tricycle and catching a ball are often not accomplished before age 3 years.

Gross motor skills and physical activity are related and stimulate reciprocally. A recent review found that among children under 5 years of age, moderate-to-vigorous physical activity was consistently associated with motor development, fitness, and bone and skeletal health [6]. The World Health Organization has recently released guidelines for physical activity among children under 5 years of age [7], emphasizing the importance of toddlers developing appropriate physical activity habits.

By 12 months of age, oral motor skills, including tongue laterality, have progressed to enable toddlers to handle increasingly complex food by chewing, moving food to the back of the oral cavity, and swallowing. Fine motor skills also advance as toddlers practice picking up and manipulating small items, such as blocks and toys. They learn to stack blocks and to color with crayons. Applied to self-feeding, toddlers progress from using their hands to using utensils, and from drinking from a cup with a protective spout to an open cup. Although the advancing skills are often accompanied by spills and messes, they add to toddlers' sense of mastery and autonomy.

Learning

Toddlers learn through 3 primary processes: observation/imitation, exploration, and play. Imitation begins within the first 72 h after birth as newborns imitate mouth openings and tongue protrusions [8]. Young children continue to learn by observing and modeling [9]. Exploration occurs through toddlers' developing sensory and motor skills, illustrated by their interest in touching, smelling, and putting things into their mouth – both food and nonfood items. Through play, toddlers practice their emerging skills, initially by touching items to experience their sensations and then by manipulating them to figure out how they can be used. By approximately 2 years of age, toddlers develop symbolic thinking and the capacity to solve problems mentally rather than exclusively through trial and error (e.g., ability to place a square block into a square hole). In Piagetian terms, by mid-toddlerhood they progress from the sensorimotor period of relying on their senses to the preoperational period of figuring out how things work or how they come apart. Applying imitation and exploration through active play enables toddlers to learn and to develop autonomy and a sense of mastery – understanding their environment through their own actions.

The desire to explore and touch is so strong that toddlers will repeatedly touch things, even if warned that the objects are dangerous or off limits. Toddlers often strive to engage in activities and touch things that they observe family members doing even if they lack the prerequisite skills. Consequently, the prevalence of unintentional injuries is high during toddlerhood. In 2018, the prevalence of deaths due to unintentional injuries among 2-year-old children in the United States (9.9/100,000) exceeded the prevalence of deaths among children aged 4–15 years more than twofold (3.9/100,000), with deaths among 3-year-old children at 6.7/100,000 [10]. It was not until children reached 16 years of age (the age when youth can obtain a driver's license) that the prevalence of deaths exceeded that of toddlers (11.4/100,000). Although toddlers are increasing in mobility, exploration, and problem-solving skills, their ability to recognize danger is not well developed, and their risk of injuries is high. Thus, toddlers require careful supervision to avoid potential hazards, often within their home.

Language

Toddlers' language skills increase along with their advancing cognitive skills. Toddlers in multilingual settings learn to understand and speak multiple languages, and most toddlers are speaking in sentences that can be understood by nonfamily members by age 3 years. Toddlers also use their language skills to engage in pretend play, often re-enacting situations that they observe in daily life. Their ability to use symbols and imagination to engage in pretend play enables toddlers to re-enact household issues or to practice make-believe interactions with others.

Advances in language include both the number of words that children understand and speak and also complex language-specific structures. Children benefit from language-rich environments, based on contingent language in which caregivers talk about what the toddler is experiencing, and build reading into daily routines. Dialogic reading, with books becoming a stimulus for turn-taking conversations between toddlers and caregivers, has been shown to promote literacy in multiple countries [11]. Dialogic reading is the basis of Reach Out and Read, a program that has been implemented globally in homes (www.reachoutandread.org).

Sleep

Sleep patterns consolidate during toddlerhood as toddlers sleep through the night with a mid-day nap and shift from cribs to beds [12]. The American Academy of Pediatrics recommends that toddlers receive 11–14 h of sleep daily with bedtime before 9:00 PM [13]. Toddlers who receive less than the recommended amount of sleep are at increased risk for excess weight gain, emotional dysregulation, impaired growth, injuries, and lower academic achievement. In addition, shortened nighttime sleep increases the likelihood of next-day sedentary behavior [14]. With the exception of sleeping, toddlers should not be sedentary or inactive for more than 1 h at a time.

Attachment and Separation Anxiety

Infants differentiate familiar from unfamiliar people and form attachment relationships with primary caregivers that continue into toddlerhood [15]. Toddlers often use attachment relationships as a "secure base" to explore new situations. That is, knowing that the attachment figure is nearby, toddlers feel secure exploring new situations. Toddlers may also experience separation anxiety and feel anxious when primary caregivers are out of sight, illustrating a lack of understanding that the separation is temporary. Separation anxiety can be stressful for toddlers and their caregivers, particularly because toddlers may also experience frustration when they are reunited with their caregivers, particularly if they are temperamentally "difficult." In most situations, separation anxiety abates as toddlers gain more sophisticated object permanence skills and comfort in dealing with novel people and situations.

Temperament refers to children's personality or behavioral style in handling situations. The 3 primary domains of temperament are "easy," "slow to warm up," and "difficult." A child with an easy temperament goes with the flow, adjusts to changes in patterns of eating, sleeping, and playing without difficulty. A child with a slow-to-warm-up temperament may be hesitant initially but slowly adapts. A child with a difficult temperament has trouble adapting to changes or new situations, and may be negative and difficult to handle. Although temperament is thought to be intrinsic in nature, caregivers can learn to manage their toddler's temperament by providing opportunities for the toddler to experience success and learn to adapt to novel or changing situations.

Autonomy and Independence

The acquisition of multiple skills, along with a desire to explore and model what they observe, contributes to toddlers' sense of autonomy. As their mobility increases, toddlers want to do things themselves, often without help from others. Effective caregivers have rules for toddlers to enhance their development, to socialize them as family members, and to protect them from potential dangers. When toddlers perceive that rules are in conflict with their independence, they experience frustration. With their need to rely on caregivers, and their limited impulse control, temper tantrums can result. Temper tantrums are difficult for toddlers and caregivers. With effective management, often by helping the toddler focus on developmentally appropriate activities, temper tantrums can be prevented. As toddlers mature and acquire more cognitive and self-regulatory skills and better impulse control, their ability to handle autonomy and independence improves, and temper tantrums can be averted.

In summary, child development is cumulative and dynamic during toddlerhood, building on skills acquired during infancy. Gross motor advances (crawling, walking, running, and climbing) enable toddlers to explore their physical environment as they engage in goal-directed behavior. Fine motor advances enable toddlers to pick up small objects, manipulate eating utensils, and self-feed. Oral motor and language developments enable toddlers to chew complex foods, to express themselves and communicate, and to negotiate. With enhanced cognition, toddlers can solve problems, recall the location of hidden objects, and play simple games. Toddler's social development includes prosocial skills, such as empathy and recognition of others' emotions, and self-regulation, such as controlling their thoughts or behavior in response to specific contexts and situations. These emerging skills bring increasing autonomy, often accompanied by impulsivity to satisfy their desires immediately. When combined with toddlers' changing nutritional needs, their increasing autonomy can present challenges to caregivers, especially during meals.

Toddler Eating Behavior

The World Health Organization recommends exclusive breastfeeding of infants until approximately 6 months of age and then transition to complementary feeding, defined as the period when breast milk alone is no longer sufficient to meet infants' nutritional requirements. Complementary feeding extends from approximately 6 to 18 months well into toddlerhood. Breastfeeding often continues in the second year as food occupies an increasingly larger proportion of toddlers' diet. Guidelines for complementary feeding have focused primarily on toddlers' nutrient requirements and advances in flavor and texture as their diet expands and begins to approximate the family diet [16].

Baby-Led Weaning

The traditional method of complementary feeding, which begins at approximately 6 months of age, is to serve purees, spoon-fed by the caregiver, and gradually increase the flavors and consistency of foods until approximately 12 months of age, when the child transitions to the family diet [17]. Baby-led weaning, introduced in England in 2008, provides softened, bite-size foods directly to the child. Children choose when and what food they will eat (from a choice of healthy options), the rhythm of the meal, and the amount of food that they will eat while primarily feeding themselves [18]. Baby-led weaning is based on presumptions that young children have the motor skills to self-feed, along with the regulatory skills to signal hunger and satiety. Caregivers play supportive, rather than direct roles, with infants often seated with the family during meals, which facilitates modeling and enables toddlers to be included in mealtime interactions.

Three recent reviews [18–20] found that baby-led weaning typically occurs in the context of the family meal, with the child consuming food that is softened and cut into bite sizes. In comparison with traditional methods of complementary feeding, baby-led weaning was positively associated with infants' self-regulation and satiety, with timing of the initiation of complementary feeding consistent with guidelines, and with adequacy of weight gain, with some evidence of overweight among the spoon-fed group and of underweight among the baby-led group. Although there were no group differences in rates of choking or micronutrient intake, there was some suggestion that the baby-led group was at higher risk of choking and of not obtaining adequate micronutrients, often because micronutrient-rich food was offered infrequently [18]. Advantages of baby-led weaning included exposure to a wide variety of food, more interaction with the food, and exploration of multiple textures. Baby-led weaning has been adopted by families in many countries, including England, New Zealand, and Brazil, for example. Evidence addressing the nutrient intake and long-term impact of baby-led weaning on children's nutrient intake and eating patterns is emerging.

Food Neophobia

Food neophobia, defined as refusal or fear to eat unfamiliar foods, is a normal developmental phase during toddlerhood that declines during childhood. From an ethological perspective, neophobia is adaptive because it protects children from novel foods that may be harmful or bitter. Food neophobia differs from selectivity or pickiness, defined as specific food preferences and dislikes, regardless of familiarity. A recent systematic review and meta-analysis of neophobia and picky eating emphasized the relevance of considering the social context and bidirectional parent-toddler aspects of feeding, including factors at the biological, child, parent, and household levels [21].

Evidence has shown that 10 or more presentations of the novel food may be necessary to overcome neophobia [21]. Food neophobia is often managed through familiarity and modeling with family members eating the novel foods. If familiarity and modeling are not effective, caregivers may remove the novel food from the toddler's diet or attempt to force the toddler to eat the novel food. Limiting the toddler's food choices denies access to healthy foods and teaches the toddler the power of refusal. Using force or pressuring techniques may in-

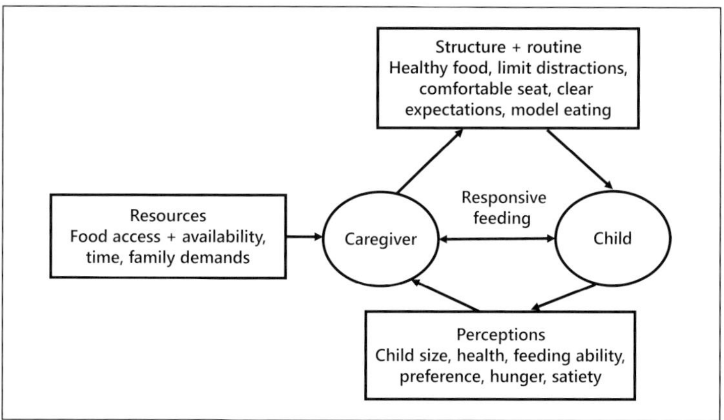

Fig. 1. Responsive feeding.

crease resistance and lead to confrontational mealtimes, particularly among children who are temperamentally difficult.

Neophobia can transition into pickiness, especially if caregivers attempt to use controlling or coercive strategies. The autonomy that toddlers have developed makes them want to be agents of their own preferences and actions [22]. They may resist food that looks or smells unfamiliar or unappealing or because they can resist. If their resistance results in conflict, a negative pattern may result whereby caregivers perceive the toddler to be resistant or picky, and they then implement maladaptive strategies. A reconceptualization of neophobia has been suggested to consider the roles and perceptions of both caregivers and toddlers, to reduce the tension in their interaction, to move away from the "picky eater" term, and to focus on caregivers' expectations of children's eating and mealtime interactions [22].

Responsive Feeding

Responsive feeding, a derivative of responsive parenting, is based on the principle that feeding young children is bidirectional and guided by toddlers' internal sense of hunger and satiety. Responsive feeding is embedded in a parenting style that includes both structure and responsivity [23]. The structure refers to caregivers' establishing routines, with consistent meal patterns, timing, context, food choices, and expected behavior (e.g., eating food, no throwing food). Distractions, such as television and other screens, are removed, and meals are coordinated with others eating to provide appropriate modeling (Fig. 1). Responsivity is guided by the caregiver's perceptions of the toddler's characteristics, including size, health, feeding skills, and especially by the toddler's signals of

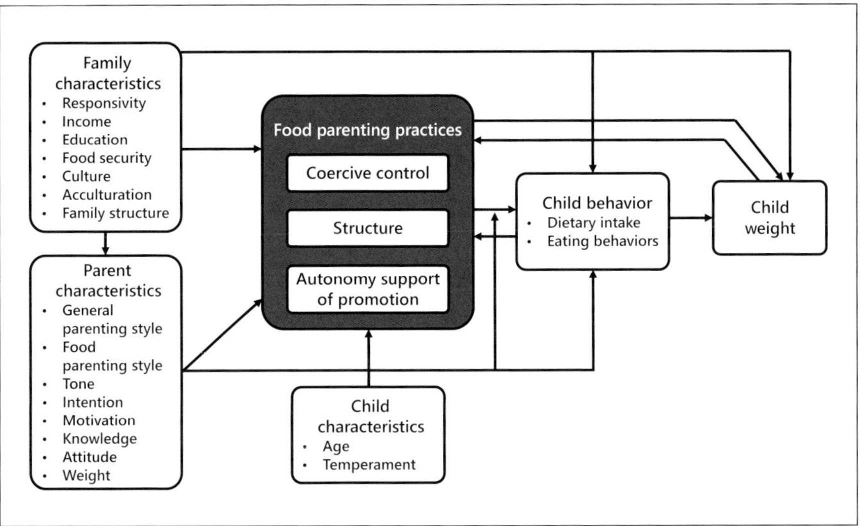

Fig. 2. Food parenting practices: coercive control, structure, and autonomy support [24].

hunger and satiety. Caregiver responses are prompt, clear, nurturant, and developmentally appropriate. When the toddler signals satiety, the caregiver ends the meal and maintains a pleasant demeanor.

A recent review identified 3 food parenting practices used with young children, including toddlers: coercive control, structure, and autonomy support (Fig. 2) [24]. Coercive control refers to controlling practices, including pressure to eat, threats, and bribes, and using food to control negative emotions. Structure refers to rules and limits, limited/guided choices, monitoring, meal- and snack time routines, modeling, food availability and accessibility, and food preparation. Autonomy support includes facilitating self-feeding, child involvement, and encouragement. The structure and autonomy support constructs are consistent with responsive feeding guidelines.

In spite of global recommendations that responsive feeding be implemented, there is no consensus on measures to be used to measure responsive feeding. A recent review identified 15 instruments developed for children from birth to 2 years of age and 28 for children aged 3–5 years [25]. Only 3 of the 43 instruments showed rigorous validation and reliability testing. Most relied on caregiver report and had not been validated against observations. There is clearly a need for a validated assessment of responsive feeding for toddlers to facilitate communication across investigations and the evaluation of intervention trials.

In summary, toddlerhood is a transitional period that can be both joyful and challenging, as children acquire new skills and assert their autonomy. Feeding is particularly challenging because there are clear expectations for caregivers to ensure that their toddlers receive adequate nutrients. Recently recognized strategies, including baby-led weaning, may facilitate the transition to complementary feeding and the family diet. However, additional research is needed to ensure that infants can feed themselves safely and acquire micro- and macronutrients required. Although neophobia is developmentally normal and typically resolves, it introduces challenges to families and can transition into pickiness. Effective parenting practices include the structure of providing healthy food and age-appropriate settings and opportunities for toddlers to feed themselves. In addition, responsive feeding requires caregivers to read toddlers' signals and to respond promptly, appropriately, and with nurturance. This pattern ensures that toddlers receive the guidance and nurturant care that is needed to develop healthy feeding behavior and emotional well-being [26].

Conflict of Interest Statement

Maureen M. Black has no conflicts of interest.

References

1 Birch LL, Davison KK: Family environmental factors influencing the developing behavioral controls of food intake and childhood overweight. Pediatr Clin 2001;48:893–907.
2 Haines J, McDonald J, O'Brien A, et al: Healthy Habits, Happy Homes: randomized trial to improve household routines for obesity prevention among preschool-aged children. JAMA Pediatr 2013;167:1072–1079.
3 Cunningham SA, Kramer MR, Narayan KV: Incidence of childhood obesity in the United States. N Engl J Med 2014;370:403–411.
4 World Health Organization: Report of the Commission on Ending Obesity. Geneva, WHO, 2016. http://www.who.int/end-childhood-obesity/en/.
5 Pan L, Blanck HM, Park S, et al: State-specific prevalence of obesity among children aged 2–4 years enrolled in the Special Supplemental Nutrition Program for Women, Infants, and Children – United States, 2010–2016. MMWR Morb Mortal Wkly Rep 2019;68:1057–1061.
6 Carson V, Lee EY, Hewitt L, et al: Systematic review of the relationships between physical activity and health indicators in the early years (0–4 years). BMC Public Health 2017;17(Suppl 5):854.
7 World Health Organization: Guidelines on Physical Activity, Sedentary Behaviour and Sleep for Children under 5 Years of Age. Geneva, WHO, 2019. https://apps.who.int/iris/handle/10665/311664.
8 Meltzoff AN, Moore MK: Newborn infants imitate adult facial gestures. Child Dev 1983;54:702–709.
9 Shimpi PM, Akhtar N, Moore C: Toddlers' imitative learning in interactive and observational contexts: the role of age and familiarity of the model. J Exp Child Psychol 2013;116:309–323.
10 Injury Prevention & Control: Data & Statistics (WISQARS™). http://www.cdc.gov/injury/wisqars/index.html (accessed Apr 18, 2020).
11 Zuckerman B, Elansary M, Needlman R: Book sharing: in-home strategy to advance early child development globally. Pediatrics 2019;143:e20182033.
12 Mindell JA, Williamson AA: Benefits of a bedtime routine in young children: sleep, development, and beyond. Sleep Med Rev 2018;40:93–108.
13 American Academy of Pediatrics: Toddlers. https://www.healthychildren.org/Eng;osh/ages-stages/toddler/Pages/default.aspx.

14 Armstrong B, Covington LB, Unick GJ, Black MM: Bidirectional effects of sleep and sedentary behavior among toddlers. J Pediatr Psychol 2019; 44:278–285.
15 Ainsworth MDS, Blehar MC, Waters E, Wall S: Patterns of Attachment: A Psychological Study of the Strange Situation. Hillsdale, Lawrence Erlbaum, 1978.
16 Rapley G, Forste R, Cameron S, et al: Baby-led weaning: a new frontier. ICAN 2015;7:77–85.
17 PAHO/WHO. Guiding Principles for Complementary Feeding of the Breastfed Child. Washington, Pan American Health Organization, 2003.
18 Gomez MS, Novaes APT, Silva JPD, et al: Baby-led weaning. An overview of the new approach to food introduction. Rev Paul Pediatr 2020; 38:e2018084.
19 Andries AL, Nevesa FS, Camposa AL, Netto MP: The bay-led weaning method (BLW) in the context of complementary feeding: a review. Rev Paul Pediatr 2018;36:353–363.
20 Brown A, Jones SW, Rowan H: Baby-led weaning: the evidence to date. Curr Nutr Rep 2017;6:148–156.
21 Cole NC, An R, Lee SY, Donovan SM: Correlates of picky eating and food neophobia in young children: a systematic review and meta-analysis. Nutr Rev 2017;75:516–532.
22 Walton K, Kuczynski L, Haycraft E, et al: Time to re-think picky eating? A relational approach to understanding picky eating. Int J Behav Nutr Phys Act 2017;14:62.
23 Black MM, Aboud F: Responsive feeding is embedded in a theoretical framework of responsive parenting. J Nutr 2011;141:490–494.
24 Vaughn AE, Ward DS, Fisher JO, et al: Fundamental constructs in food parenting practices: a content map to guide future research. Nutr Rev 2016;74:98–117.
25 Heller RL, Mobley AR: Instruments assessing parental responsive feeding in children ages birth to 5 years: a systematic review. Appetite 2019; 138:23–51.
26 Verhage CL, Gillebaart M, van der Veek SMC, Vereijken CMJL: The relation between family meals and health of infants and toddlers: a review. Appetite 2018;127:97–109.

Published online: November 9, 2020

Black MM, Singhal A, Hillman CH (eds): Building Future Health and Well-Being of Thriving Toddlers and Young Children. Nestlé Nutr Inst Workshop Ser. Basel, Karger, 2020, vol 95, pp 12–22 (DOI: 10.1159/000511519)

Global Landscape of Nutrient Inadequacies in Toddlers and Young Children

Alison L. Eldridge Elizabeth A. Offord

Nestlé Research, Nestlé Institute of Health Sciences, Lausanne, Switzerland

Abstract

Toddlers and young children need an adequate and diverse diet to provide all of the nutrients required for optimal growth and development. Unfortunately, inadequate intake of vitamins and minerals is still identified by the World Health Organization (WHO) as a major public health threat for young children. Organizations like the WHO and the World Bank focus primarily on iron, zinc, vitamin A, and iodine for children ≤5 years of age in low-income countries. In addition to the data from these organizations, individual-level food consumption surveys are needed to provide a fuller picture of food and nutrient intakes. Where studies are available, intakes of dietary fiber and vitamin D are generally below recommendations for toddlers and young children. Other nutrient gaps differ by country and are related to food availability and local dietary habits. For example, young children in the US regularly consume dairy products, and <10% fall below recommendations for calcium intake compared to 2- to 4-year-old toddlers in the Philippines where dairy food consumption is low, and 66–84% fall below calcium recommendations. Dietary intake studies can help to identify the foods and beverages most relevant to alleviate nutrient gaps and improve dietary intakes of toddlers and young children around the world.

Introduction

Toddlers and young children need an adequate and diverse diet to provide all of the nutrients they require to support optimal growth and development. Unfortunately, undernutrition, growing rates of overweight and obesity, and inadequate intakes of vitamins and minerals are still identified as major public health threats for young children by the World Health Organization (WHO) [1]. For micronutrients, the WHO, UNICEF, and the World Bank focus primarily on iron, zinc, vitamin A, and iodine. Global monitoring shows that the combination of anemia rates, along with vitamin A deficiency and stunting, lead to an "alarmingly high" hidden hunger index in certain regions of the world, particularly sub-Saharan Africa and South Asia [2].

In addition to the global data from these organizations, individual-level food consumption surveys are needed to provide a fuller picture of food and nutrient intakes in different countries. However, these surveys are generally available in higher-income countries and are less common in low- and middle-income countries in regions such as Africa, Eastern Europe, and Southeast Asia [3]. Even among European countries with a food consumption survey, not all collect data on toddlers and young children [4]. National surveys in the US (National Health and Nutrition Examination Survey, NHANES) and Australia (National Nutrition and Physical Activity Survey, NNPAS) start only from the age of 2 years. Some national surveys also lack data on the full complement of nutrients required in the diet.

It is our aim, therefore, to evaluate what is known about the nutritional challenges and inadequacies facing toddlers across the world. With many sources of data, each one helps to build our knowledge by telling a different piece of the story. We will evaluate the information provided from each type of study and explore similarities and differences in the nutritional gaps of young children globally.

Monitoring Young Child Growth and Weight

The WHO, UNICEF, and the World Bank monitor several measures of growth and weight in children under 5 years of age globally [1, 5]. These measures help to identify and track problems of inadequate (wasting, stunting, and underweight) and excess nutrition (overweight and obesity), and because the measures are standardized, they also allow for comparisons across countries and over time. They are used by the WHO and UNICEF in collaboration with the Food and Agriculture Organization (FAO), the International Fund for Agricultural Development (IFAD), and the World Food Program (WFP) to monitor

Table 1. Percentage of children 12–23 months of age achieving minimum dietary diversity, minimum feedi frequency, and minimum acceptable diet scores by UNICEF region

Region	Children who achieved the minimum score (range), %		
	minimum dietary diversity score[1]	minimum meal frequency[2]	minimum acceptable diet[3]
East Asia and Pacific	47.1 (25.6–71.5)	71.3 (44.3–93.7)	35.1 (14.2–60.9)
South Asia	39.0 (18.1–78.0)	62.7 (39.0–74.7)	28.4 (11.9–54.1)
Eastern Europe and Central Asia	62.6 (29.8–92.4)	74.8 (43.3–97.7)	49.0 (12.5–85.7)
Middle East and North Africa	48.1 (25.2–68.6)	69.3 (52.5–90.2)	36.2 (18.2–60.7)
Eastern and Southern Africa	28.8 (14.4–48.4)	41.4 (12.1–83.6)	14.5 (7.2–36.0)
West and Central Africa	21.1 (6.5–40.0)	42.5 (23.1–63.9)	11.2 (2.6–23.8)
Latin America and the Caribbean	64.4 (19.8–87.7)	72.9 (34.4–89.4)	50.1 (10.1–71.1)

The minimum dietary diversity consists of 8 food groups: (i) breast milk; (ii) grains, roots, and tubers; (iii) legum and nuts; (iv) dairy products (infant formula, milk, yogurt, and cheese); (v) flesh foods (meat, fish, poultry, a liver/organ meats); (vi) eggs; (vii) vitamin-A-rich fruits and vegetables; and (viii) other fruits and vegetables.
[1] Percent of children who received ≥5 foods of the 8 food groups during the previous day.
[2] Percent of children who received a minimum meal frequency defined as 3 times solid, semisolid, or soft foo for breastfed children, and 4 times solid, semisolid, or soft foods and/or milk feeds for nonbreastfed children.
[3]Percent of children who received a minimum acceptable diet defined as those who had at least the minimu dietary diversity and the minimum meal frequency during the previous day (breastfed children) and those w received at least 2 milk feedings and had at least the minimum dietary diversity not including milk feedings a the minimum meal frequency during the previous day (nonbreastfed children).

50.1% in Latin America and the Caribbean. These assessments are qualitative, not quantitative, so specific estimates of energy and nutrient intakes are not possible with these instruments.

Dietary Intake Surveys

Detailed data on food and nutrient intakes and dietary patterns in young children require other methods and sources of data. National individual-level dietary intake surveys generally use multiple-day interviewer-assisted 24-h recalls or detailed diet diaries to estimate nutrient intakes and evaluate food patterns, but even with comprehensive surveys, not all include intakes of young children. For example, Huybrechts et al. [3] identified 39 national individual-level food consumption surveys globally, but less than half included children under the age of 5 years. Out of 18 countries with national surveys in Europe (2000–2016), only two-thirds reported energy and nutrient intakes for children ≤5 years [4].

Other large-scale surveys, such as the Feeding Infants and Toddlers Study (FITS) [11] and the South East Asian Nutrition Survey (SEANUTS) [12], in-

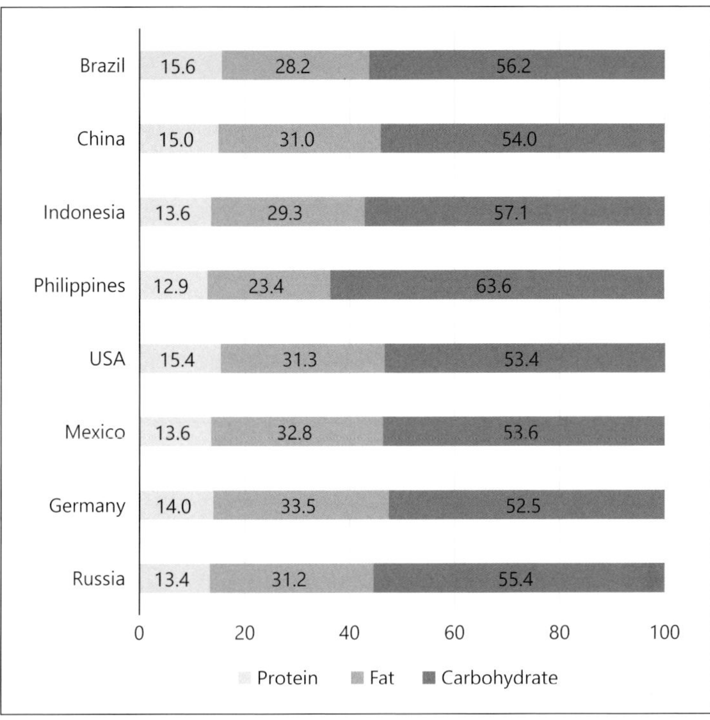

Fig. 1. Macronutrient distribution in toddlers and young children in selected countries.

clude detailed dietary assessments of young children. FITS is a cross-sectional study in the US started in 2002, with subsequent surveys collected in 2008 and 2016. FITS provides comprehensive dietary intake data for infants, toddlers, and young children from birth up to the age of 4 years. A similar approach was used in China for the Maternal Infant Nutrition Growth (MING) study [13, 14]. FITS has also been used as a model to analyze national survey data on toddlers and young children from other countries, including Mexico [15, 16], Russia [17], and the Philippines [18]. SEANUTS was conducted in Indonesia, Malaysia, Thailand, and Vietnam, and included data from children 6 months to 12 years of age; data from Indonesia are included here as an example [19]. Survey data from a multicenter study in 9 cities in Brazil [20] and nationwide samples of German toddlers [21, 22] are also included for comparison purposes.

When looking at the detailed dietary intake studies, we find wide ranges in energy intakes for 2- to 3-year-old children, with lower intakes in the Philippines (839 kcal/day) [18] and Indonesia (965 kcal/day) [19], and higher intakes in Brazil (1,650 kcal/day) [20], the USA (1,397 kcal/day) [23], and Mexico (1,367 kcal/

day) [16]. Energy intakes were intermediate in children 2–3 years old from Russia (1,243 kcal/day) [17], Germany (1,075 kcal/day) [21], and China (1,189 kcal/day) [13]. Energy intakes corresponded to higher rates of stunting in the Philippines, and higher rates of overweight and obesity in Brazil, North America, and Europe [2]. The distribution of energy from protein, fat, and carbohydrates also differs by country, with higher carbohydrate and lower fat intakes in Southeast Asia (Fig. 1).

Dietary fiber and vitamin D intakes are generally below recommendations for toddlers and young children, though vitamin D is not reported for every country (Table 2). Other nutrient gaps differ by country and are related to food availability and local dietary habits. For example, US children 2–4 years old regularly consume dairy products [24], and <10% (6.4% of children 24–35 months old and 9.2% of those 36–47 months old) fall below recommendations for calcium intakes [23]. In contrast, in the Philippines and Indonesia, where consumption of dairy foods is rare, 66–84% of children 2–4 years old fall below calcium recommendations [18, 19]. For vitamin E, we see relatively low levels of inadequacy in China (6%), moderate inadequacy for the US (32%) and Germany (43%), and high levels of inadequacy for the Philippines (>90%). Iron intakes are below recommendations for the majority of children in Indonesia (83%), the Philippines (75%), and Russia (64%), in contrast to those living in the USA, Mexico, and Brazil, where <5% are below recommendations.

In addition to nutrient intakes, detailed food consumption surveys can be analyzed to gain insights into dietary patterns, including amounts consumed from different food groups [24], food sources of energy and nutrients [14, 15, 18], or patterns of consumption, such as milk [17, 25] and beverage consumption [26, 27]. For example, we have been able to demonstrate the important role that fortified milk plays in the diet of young children in the Philippines [25] and have modeled the impact of fortified milk in reaching dairy recommendations in China [28]. These types of analyses provide insights into why certain nutrients may be below (or above) recommended levels and help to better understand the impact of potential changes to dietary habits for children in different countries of the world.

Conclusions

Several important sources of data on nutrition status and dietary intakes are available globally. International monitoring from the WHO, UNICEF, and the World Bank provides information on growth rates (stunting, wasting, underweight, overweight, and obesity) in children under the age of 5 years, and iden-

Table 2. Dietary fiber and micronutrient inadequacies (mean values per day and percentages below estimated average requirements [EAR]) in young children from selected countries

Country	Fibers, g/day	Vitamin A		Vitamin C		Vitamin D		Vitamin E		Calcium		Iron		Zinc	
		μg	% <EAR	mg	% <EAR	μg	% <EAR	mg	% <EAR	mg	% <EAR	mg	% <EAR	mg	% <EAR
EAR/AI	19	210		13		10		5		500		3.0		2.5	
Brazil [20] 2–3 years	15.5	924	0.7	312.9	0	5.3	93.6	5.4	15.1	807	12.6	13.4	0.4	9.7	0
China [13] 24–35 months	5.9	587	19.7	76.1	34.6	–	–	12.4	6.0	646	48.4	15.2	12.7	7.6	–
Indonesia [19] 2–4.9 years	–	467	78.6	37.7	83.5	–	–	–	–	412	79.6	5.8	82.7	–	–
Philippines [18] 24–35 months	3.5	365	41	23.1	35	2.3	–	2.0	>90	421	66	5.2	75	5.0	46
USA [23] 24–35 months	12.0	603	4.2	80	0	6.8	80	7.3	32	961	6.4	11.0	4.1	7.7	0.4
Mexico [16][1] 24–47 months	14.2	595	3.5	107.1	0.4	8.4	71.4	13.6	12.0	814	21.6	11.0	2.9	8.7	0.3
Germany [21, 22] 25–35 months	12.3	646	25.4	68.6	–	1.1	–	5.7	43.2	609	35.2	6.3	12.5	5.1	7.4
Russia [17] 24–35 months	7.9	357	65.2	33.5	67.8	–	–	–	–	554	78.8	8.6	63.7	–	–

EAR, estimated average requirement; AI, adequate intake level (National Academies of Sciences, Engineering, and Medicine 2019; https://doi.org/10.17226/25353); EARs are available for all vitamins and minerals listed; AI is used for fiber. Inadequacy was compared to US EAR values, except for Indonesia and Russia, which were compared to their locally recommended dietary allowances.

[1] Includes Piernas et al. [16] and unpublished data from ENSANUT (Encuesta Nacional de Salud y Nutrición) 2012.

tifies countries where young children are at risk for deficiencies in vitamin A, iron, zinc, and iodine. The WHO has also created simple qualitative diet quality indicators that can be assessed using DHS and MICS surveys to help understand the risk for inadequate dietary intakes. These indicators are used as a basis for policy decisions and program interventions but are not designed to provide quantitative intake data on energy or nutrients. For quantitative data, national-level detailed dietary intake studies are required to complement global monitoring of nutritional issues by the WHO and the World Bank.

National surveys provide population estimates of energy and nutrient intakes. By comparing with reference values, they can be used to identify the percentage of children and other population groups at risk for inadequate or excess intake. While many high-quality national surveys exist, there is still a gap in knowledge. For example, not all countries conduct quantitative national-level dietary intake studies. In those that do, not all studies include young children. Although food composition databases are constantly improving, there are discussions regarding the harmonization of nutrient reference standards [29] underway, and the European Food Safety Authority (EFSA) has put in place a common framework for conducting dietary intake surveys across Europe, called the EU MENU project [30]. However, there are still marked differences in the quality of food composition databases and methods used to conduct and analyze comprehensive national nutrition surveys around the world. Improving the quality of food composition data, harmonizing nutrient reference standards, and using more consistent methodology will all help to improve our understanding of nutrient intakes and dietary patterns. High-quality dietary intake information for young children is still needed to help identify the foods and beverages most relevant to alleviate nutrient gaps and improve dietary intakes of toddlers and young children.

Using the data we have, we can see that child growth issues like stunting still affect approximately one-third of children <5 years of age in Southern Asia, Central and Eastern Africa, and parts of Oceania, while overweight is rising in all regions of the world. Rates of anemia, vitamin A, and zinc deficiency are also highest in South Asia and Central African countries. The DHS and MICS show that fewer than 15% of children 12–23 months old in Central African countries and less than 30% in South Asian countries reach the minimum acceptable diet score.

A deeper dive into the nutrient intakes from quantitative national nutrition surveys shows wide ranges in nutrient intakes for 2- to 3-year-old toddlers from Brazil, China, Indonesia, the Philippines, the USA, Mexico, Germany, and Russia. We saw generally low fiber and vitamin D intakes in the countries presented here, and wide variability in the percentage of young children with low intakes for vitamins A, C, and E, and for calcium, iron, and zinc. Understanding dietary patterns can provide additional insight into the food-related causes of these inadequate intakes and help to define appropriate targets for improving nutrient intakes.

Conflict of Interest Statement

The authors, Alison L. Eldridge and Elizabeth A. Offord, are employees of Nestlé Research, Vers-chez-les-Blanc, Lausanne, Switzerland (Société des Produits Nestlé S.A.). Nestlé Research funded FITS in the USA, analysis of the MING study in China, and analysis of national nutrition survey data for Mexico, the Philippines, and Russia.

References

1 World Health Organization: Malnutrition. 16 Feb 2018. https://www.who.int/news-room/fact-sheets/detail/malnutrition (accessed Feb 2, 2020).
2 Ritchie H, Roser M: Our World in Data (https://ourworldindata.org/). Micronutrient Deficiency 2020 (https://ourworldindata.org/micronutrient-deficiency). Obesity 2020 (https://ourworldindata.org/obesity). Share of Children Who Are Stunted, 2016 (https://ourworldindata.org/grapher/child-stunting-ihme) (accessed Feb 3, 2020).
3 Huybrechts I, Aglago EK, Mullee A, et al: Global comparison of national individual food consumption surveys as a basis for health research and integration in national health surveillance programmes. Proc Nutr Soc 2017;76:549–567.
4 Rippin HL, Hutchinson J, Jewell J, et al: Child and adolescent nutrient intakes from current national dietary surveys of European populations. Nutr Res Rev 2018;32:38–69.
5 United Nations Children's Fund (UNICEF), World Health Organization, the World Bank: Levels and Trends in Child Malnutrition: Key Findings of the 2019 Edition of the Joint Child Malnutrition Estimates. Geneva, World Health Organization, 2019.
6 FAO, IFAD, UNICEF, WFP, WHO: The State of Food Security and Nutrition in the World 2019. Safeguarding against Economic Slowdowns and Downturns. Rome, FAO, 2019.
7 World Health Organization: Guideline: Fortification of Food-Grade Salt with Iodine for the Prevention and Control of Iodine Deficiency Disorders. Geneva, WHO, 2014.
8 World Health Organization: Global Nutrition Monitoring Framework: Operational Guidance for Tracking Progress in Meeting Targets for 2025. Geneva, World Health Organization, 2017.
9 Kennedy G, Ballard T, Dop M: Guidelines for Measuring Household and Individual Dietary Diversity. Rome, Nutrition and Consumer Protection Division, FAO, 2013.
10 United Nations Children's Fund, Division of Data, Analysis, Planning, and Monitoring: Global UNICEF Global Databases: Infant and Young Child Feeding: Minimum Acceptable Diet, Minimum Diet Diversity, Minimum Meal Frequency. New York, UNICEF, 2019.
11 Eldridge AL: FITS and KNHS overview: methodological challenges in dietary intake data collection among infants, toddlers and children in selected countries; in Henry CJ, Nicklas TA, Nicklaus S (eds): Nurturing a Health Generation of Children: Research Gaps and Opportunities. Nestlé Nutrition Institute Workshop Series. Basel, Karger, 2019, vol 91, pp 69–78.
12 Schaafsma A, Deurenberg P, Calame W, et al, SEANUTS Study Group: Design of the South East Asian Nutrition Survey (SEANUTS): a four-country multistage cluster design study. Br J Nutr 2013;110:S2–S10.
13 Chen C, Denney L, Zheng Y, et al: Nutrient intakes of infants and toddlers from maternal and child care centres in urban areas of China, based on one 24 h dietary recall. BMC Nutr 2015;1:23.
14 Wang H, Denney L, Zheng Y, et al: Food sources of energy and nutrients in the diets of infants and toddlers in urban areas of China, based on one 24-hour dietary recall. BMC Nutr 2015;1:19.
15 Denney L, Afeiche MC, Eldridge AL, Villalpando-Carrion S: Food sources of energy and nutrients in infants, toddlers, and young children from the Mexican National Health and Nutrition Survey 2012. Nutrients 2017;9:494.

16 Piernas C, Miles DR, Deming DM, et al: Estimating usual intakes mainly affects the micronutrient distribution among infants, toddlers and preschoolers from the 2012 Mexican National Health and Nutrition Survey. Public Health Nutr 2016; 19:1017–1026.
17 Keshabyants EE, Martinchik AN, Safronova AI, et al: The practice of feeding infants during the second and third years of life in Russia (analysis of the statistics of the Federal State Statistics Service Rosstat, 2013) (in Russian). Vopr Det Dietol (Pediatric Nutrition) 2017;15:11–17.
18 Denney L, Angeles-Agdeppa I, Capanzana MV: Nutrient intakes and food sources of Filipino infants, toddlers and young children are inadequate: findings from the National Nutrition Survey 2013. Nutrients 2018;10:1730.
19 Sandjaja S, Budiman B, Harahap H, et al: Food consumption and nutritional and biochemical status of 0.5–12-year-old Indonesian children: the SEANUTS study. Br J Nutr 2013;110:S11–S20.
20 Bueno MB, Fisberg RM, Maximino P, et al: Nutritional risk among Brazilian children 2–6 years old: a multicenter study. Nutrition 2013;29:405–410.
21 Hilbig A, Drossard C, Kersting M, Alexy U: Nutrient adequacy and associated factors in a nationwide sample of German toddlers. J Pediatr Gastroenterol Nutr 2015;61:130–137.
22 Hilger J, Goerig T, Weber P, et al: Micronutrient intake in healthy toddlers: a multinational perspective. Nutrients 2015;7:6938–6955.
23 Bailey RL, Catellier DJ, Jun S, et al: Total usual nutrient intakes of US children (under 48 months): findings from the Feeding Infants and Toddlers Study (FITS) 2016. J Nutr 2018;148: 1557S–1566S.
24 Welker EB, Jacquier EF, Catellier DJ, et al: Room for improvement remains in food consumption patterns of young children aged 2–4 years. J Nutr 2018;148;1536S–1546S.
25 Mak T-N, Angeles-Agdeppa I, Tassy M, et al: Contribution of milk beverages to nutrient adequacy of young children and preschool children in the Philippines. Nutrients 2020;12:E392.
26 Afeiche MC, Villalpando-Carrión S, Reidy KC, et al: Many infants and young children are not compliant with Mexican and international complementary feeding recommendations for milk and other beverages. Nutrients 2018;10:E466.
27 Kay MC, Welker EB, Jacquier EF, Story MT: Beverage consumption patterns among infants and young children (0–47.9 months): data from the Feeding Infants and Toddlers Study, 2016. Nutrients 2018;10:E825.
28 Zhang J, Wang D, Zhang Y: Patterns of the consumption of young children formula in Chinese children aged 1–3 years and implications for nutrient intake. Nutrients 2020;12:1672.
29 National Academies of Sciences, Engineering, and Medicine: Global Harmonization of Methodological Approaches to Nutrient Intake Recommendations: Proceedings of a Workshop in Brief. Washington, National Academies Press, 2018.
30 European Food Safety Authority: Guidance on the EU Menu methodology. EFSA J 2014;12:3944.

Published online: November 6, 2020

Black MM, Singhal A, Hillman CH (eds): Building Future Health and Well-Being of Thriving Toddlers and Young Children. Nestlé Nutr Inst Workshop Ser. Basel, Karger, 2020, vol 95, pp 23–32 (DOI: 10.1159/000511509)

Nutrition Related-Practices in Brazilian Preschoolers: Identifying Challenges and Addressing Barriers

Mauro Fisberg[a, b] Lais Duarte Batista[c]

[a]Center of Nutrology and Feeding Difficulties, Instituto Pensi, Fundação José Luiz Egydio Setúbal, Hospital Infantil Sabará, São Paulo, Brazil; [b]Department of Medicine, Federal University of Sao Paulo, (UNIFESP), São Paulo, Brazil; [c]Department of Nutrition, School of Public Health, University of São Paulo (FPS/USP), São Paulo, Brazil

Abstract

Over the past decades, Brazil has faced important challenges regarding the nutrition of toddlers. Changes in dietary intake and feeding habits switched the scenario from undernutrition to increased rates of overweight and obesity. Determinants related to that issue involve the disparity in income distribution, the structure of food production and access, and the role of programs and policies, mostly related to its historical context. The feeding of Brazilian toddlers is characterized by low consumption of fruits, vegetables, and fiber, and high and early intake of fried foods, salty snacks, and sugar. Skipping important meals, e.g., breakfast, and poor snacking habits are also important practices related to excess weight. Integrated actions aiming to establish healthy eating habits in children must involve families, schools, governments, and food industry. Exploring the variety of fruits and vegetables available in the country helps to provide a healthy nutrition environment. Increasing the availability of nutrient-dense foods in the home environment improves the quality of food directed to children. Improving children's diet quality goes beyond promoting nutrition education. A favorable environment enabling to translate intentions into practice is essential, and it involves a multisectoral and an integrated framework with individual modifications and political interventions.

Introduction

Adequate nutrition in early life stages is an aspect of vital importance that affects growth, development, and health. However, it is still challenging to provide nutrient-rich diets and adequate feeding during childhood. Knowing the relevance of good nutrition is still not enough to establish healthy eating habits. A key strategy to overcome this problem involves identifying and facing barriers related to child nutrition all over the world. To discuss challenges and opportunities in different contexts and realities, we wanted to contribute some aspects related to the situation of eating habits in Brazilian toddlers.

A Historical Pathway throughout Nutrition in Brazil

The context of nutrition in Brazil is parallel to its history and linked to some aspects of Brazilian development. The disparity in income distribution, the structure of food production and access, and the role of programs and policies that attempt to modify the nutritional context are factors significantly related to the issue of malnutrition in the country.

For centuries, Brazil was a colony following the European settlement, which was reflected by its national economy. The circumstances of segregation during its expansion brought social differences with contemporary impacts on its population. In contrast to other Latin-American countries, African slaves and not natives were the most import labor workers in the colonial period, and mixing with European settlers was intense. Natives were segregated outside the cities and lived in very poor conditions, not used frequently as slaves. The migration history also played an important role in Brazilian cuisine and food patterns. The mix of native and immigrant influences coming from Africa, Europe, and later Asia reflected the country's food habits and the regional differences in Brazilian feeding. African descendants and indigenous natives, for example, are two historically important cultures for the country's development. Nevertheless, even nowadays, these groups are the ones that mostly live in a socially vulnerable situation. The racial inequality in the population income aggravates the existence of malnutrition. In 2018, a total of 60% of the overall population received less than the minimum wage. White workers received, on average, about 75% more than blacks and browns [1].

Income influences the nutritional status of toddlers through various mechanisms. Poverty affects toddlers' growth and development because it forces people to live in environments prone to diseases without clean water or adequate sanitation. Besides, low-income families tend to have less access to fresh food due to lack of its affordability in terms of income and its availability in their home environment.

The demographic scenario is another determinant for food access and availability apart from exacerbating social and health disparities. Brazil is a country of continental proportions and, therefore, qualified to stand as one of the largest food producers in the world. It is a leader in the global market and exportation of commodities such as coffee, soybeans, corn, sugar cane, cocoa, and beef. Additionally, due to its biodiversity and tropical climate, a large variety of fruits and vegetables can be cultivated. On the other hand, however, the dimensional territory did not develop equally in all regions. There is a concentration of income and resources in some areas, while other places struggle to meet the basic needs. Most of the food products are exported, while the distribution and access to affordable healthy food vary disparately across the country.

Developmental challenges such as poverty, social inequalities, and food insecurity were determinants in the scenario of malnutrition in Brazil. For many decades, children undernutrition was a key situation in the country, and the number of malnourished children was high. Inadequate intake of essential nutrients, because of poor eating habits, is one of the main unresolved problems in the country even today. A multicenter study found a high prevalence of inadequate intake, i.e., below the recommendations for fibers, calcium, and vitamins D and E in children aged 2–6 years. On the other hand, sodium intake was higher than the upper intake level in 90% of children younger than 4 years [2].

Policy initiatives to improve the dietary habits of children, especially those from socially vulnerable families, were developed in Brazil particularly in the last 2 decades. The established programs and policies attempted to tackle the structural causes of hunger, poverty, and malnutrition. A reference initiative in the country is the *Bolsa Família* Program (small amounts of money for needed families) that aims to supplement income and improve health and educational opportunities. The program was part of "The Zero Hunger Strategy," which incorporated a range of existing initiatives to guarantee universal access to quality food, based in a multisectoral framework [3].

However, increasing income did not seem to be enough to solve the problem of malnutrition and overcome the challenges in Brazilian nutrition history. Families in socially vulnerable situations did not necessarily turn access to financial resources into healthy food acquisitions. Data from the last "Research of Family Budget" *(Pesquisa de Orçamentos Familiares* – POF*)* showed a tendency to increase food consumption outside the home with increased income as well as the intake of some unhealthy foods, such as soft drinks and fast foods [4]. Instead of healthier food choices, and the inclusion of fruits and vegetables in their diets, these families seem to choose food items that are extensively consumed by higher strata of society. These vulnerable communities are also exposed to higher rates of violence and discrimination, with a built environment that is not conducive to physical activity practice. There are fewer parks and sidewalks, and there is less open space. As a result, low-income communities tend to have higher rates of obesity. This context of poor diet quality and inadequate feeding and lifestyle habits had contributed to the nutritional transition in the country. There is an increase in overweight and obesity rates in people at all income levels, which is paralleled with important nutrient deficiencies, in a hidden hunger condition. A different context facing the historically unsolved problem in the country is malnutrition.

Current Challenges regarding the Feeding of Brazilian Toddlers

Even with efforts in different sectors and contexts, overweight and obesity rates in children are still rising, and feeding and lifestyle practices are far from those recommended. Where did we fail? Why did the initiatives and strategies not work? Some specific actions in the country, but with discreet results, include programs aimed at combating malnutrition and hunger. Currently, the main problem is the lack of a well-established and multisectoral policy to tackle obesity that goes beyond discussions and takes effective actions.

Among the initiatives in the country, we can highlight the iron and folate fortification. Due to high rates of iron and folic acid deficiencies, since 2002 food fortification with these two micronutrients to all wheat and maize flours industrialized in Brazil is mandatory. However, this is not an individual strategy but a generalized fortification. Besides, there is no follow-up or surveillance of this initiative [5]. Considering that wheat and maize flours are mainly used in bread, cake, and cookie industry, the strategy is not in accordance with the promotion of universal healthy eating habits. Even with the increase in pasta and whole bread at some socioeconomic levels, without the application of other strategies such as formula milk and follow-up formulas after weaning, anemia rates rise. Complementary feeding of toddlers is expected to present a food pattern based on fresh foods such as fruits and vegetables. Therefore, in order to be efficient in overcoming hidden hunger and micronutrient deficiencies in this age group, this initiative may increase the consumption of high energy-dense and nutrition-poor foods, which are related to increased rates of overweight and obesity.

The Brazilian National School Feeding Program *(Programa Nacional de Alimentação Escolar – PNAE)* is one of the largest initiatives in school feeding in the world. However, due to the country's complexities and its large territory, schoolers are not feeding equally, and the program strategy has not worked

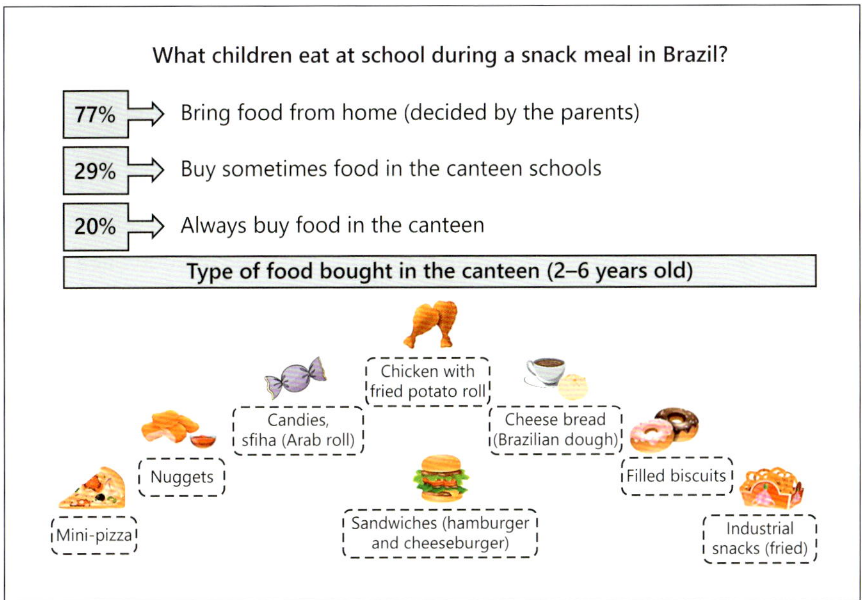

Fig. 1. Food patterns in Brazilian schools.

properly. The program is funded by the federal government and complemented with funds from municipalities and states. In Brazil, the discrepancy in development, income, and regional food availability might reflect the quality of foods purchased and, consequently, the meals served to children. Besides, Brazil has a dual educational system with private and public schools. In private schools, students usually purchase their food in the cafeterias or bring it from home. Therefore, the availability of adequate food options at school is an important barrier. The availability of several products of low nutritional content such as candies, sweet snacks, artificial juice, and soft drinks is still a reality in the school settings. Restrictions without awareness of healthy habits tend to exacerbate this trade in an uncontrolled way. To provide adequate feeding to schoolers around the country, both the educational system and families are important actors (Fig. 1).

Because this initiative does not contemplate children in preschool age, effective and pertinent participation of the family is even more needed for the feeding of toddlers. The composition of snacks, especially those served at home, is important because they are opportunities for adequate nutritional support for this age group. A study with mothers of >1,000 children aged 4–6 years from all regions of the country showed that Brazilian preschool children have the intermediate snacking habit. Positively, the fruit group was frequent in 98.8% of the snack compositions. The compositions of the morning and afternoon snacks were similar, mostly containing fruits, cookies, and yogurts. However, the afternoon snack proved to be more caloric and with more frequent intake of foods high in added sugars and of nutrient-poor content, such as candies, ice cream, and chocolates [6].

Habits involving complementary feeding are also among the families' responsibilities. There is an early and high intake of inadequate food choices, especially added sugar, sweets, biscuits, and candies, in Brazilian toddlers [7]. Most children receive cow's milk prematurely as a substitute for breast milk, which is consumed by approximately 80% of children aged 12–60 months in a national survey. In the same age group, infant formulas were consumed by less than 1% of the children [8]. Even with milk substitutes specific to the needs of toddlers, families, especially those in a vulnerable situation, cannot always afford it. In the context of children with feeding difficulties, the reality is even worse. There is an excessive daily protein intake from milk-based supplements, which tends to reduce the consumption of non-milk-based foods. Milk intake alone provided 80–138% of daily protein needs in children with feeding difficulties below 8 years of age [9]. This may result in important nutrient deficiencies, e.g., in iron, vitamin A, and fiber. The permissive parenting style has consequences not only on food patterns of toddlers but also on their eating habits. Skipping breakfast, poor snacking habits, inadequate meal timing, and lack of active participation in children feeding are important consequences in the overweight and obesity context.

Concomitant with advances in technology, early exposure to electronic devices is a worrying practice during toddler feeding. Associated with permissive parenting, the use of TVs, tablets, and cell phones has been employed as a controlling tool during mealtime. This practice affects the child's capacity to self-limit the portion sizes in addition to the development of inadequate eating habits that can affect later life. Strict strategies in the school environment are not sufficient to support healthy habits if children derive from a deficient home condition. In addition, early exposure to unhealthy food marketing can influence children's diets. The ineffective control of the government tackling aggressive marketing towards children is another barrier to the promotion of healthy feeding habits in Brazilian toddlers.

Due to the multidimensional context of the challenges, initiatives designed to promote adequate nutrition to children should be based on a framework aiming to modify families, schools, and obesogenic environments.

Opportunities to Enhance Toddlers' Feeding

Family Level

The home environment is an important space with a range of opportunities for toddlers' feeding. A potential intervention is the concept of *Nurturing Children's Healthy Eating*, a family-centered approach that recognizes the pivotal role of families in promoting and supporting children's healthy eating habits. It presents key strategies that encourage and support adequate eating practices among children. A positive parenting style avoids food restriction and encourages children's role in food choices and self-control of portion sizes. A healthy home food environment promotes the accessibility of children to appropriate foods. Positive eating practices that stimulate regular family meals, children cooking skills, and pleasure to eat are important implementations at the family level [10].

Based on the previously stated challenges, some meals play a fundamental role in promoting healthier eating habits. Toddles' breakfast, which consists mainly of milk or dairy products with chocolate flavor, is usually inadequate or incomplete. A strategy to increase the intake of other nutrients and food groups usually deficient in toddles' feeding is to use milk only as a basic ingredient of breakfast to be supplemented with fruits and cereals. Intermediate snacks are other relevant meals commonly inadequate in toddlers' eating habits. Families should invest more time, organization, and planning of their meals ahead. Dinnertime could be used as a moment to set a positive example and encourage healthy-eating socialization, i.e., a time when families have the potential to create a regular meal pattern with children and spend more time together.

Parents and caregivers should play their role of responsibility in toddlers' feeding and especially provide a healthy home environment, not be permissive regarding inadequate eating practices, such as the use of electronic devices during mealtime, and be a model of positive parenting and show active participation. We do emphasize that Brazil has one of the highest rates of using of electronic devices in small children.

School Setting

School settings are another excellent space for interventions aimed to modify food habits. Promoting nutrition education should not be a single intervention in exploring all the potential of the school environment. These initiatives must be concomitant with the promotion of activities as part of the school curriculum in a multidimensional context directed at parents, students, education professionals, and cookers.

Even if meals are served as part of the school feeding program, healthy items, such as fruits and vegetables, should be provided on a daily basis. These products

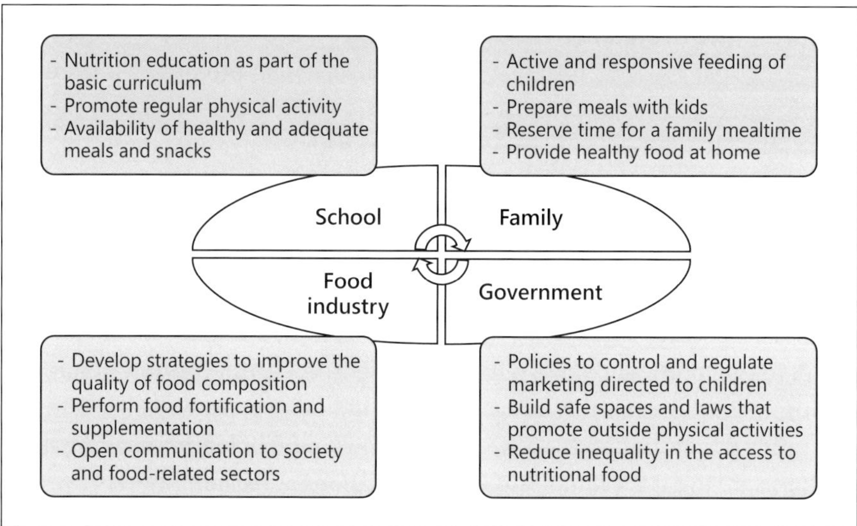

Fig. 2. Multisectoral division of responsibilities to promote healthy feeding habits in children.

have to be part of the children's food patterns and not the exception, such as occasional activities like the *Fruit Day at School.* The implementation of rules or legislation restricting unhealthy products sold in canteens is not enough to encourage the adoption of healthy habits. Children should be educated regarding healthy habits and not being exposed to inadequate food items in this environment. It is worthless to control school selling of some goods if they are available at the school doors or in close vicinity.

We should still consider the school as a space where children are educated to be conscious of adequate habits. This awareness can be unconsciously transmitted to the home environment, where children will act as a mentor in promoting healthy eating practices from school to other settings.

Obesogenic Environment

An integrated approach directed to improve toddlers' feeding includes the modification of obesogenic environment. The food industry should be even more committed to providing high-quality and nutrient-rich foods. There is a need for discussing the mandatory decrease in ingredients such as sugar and sodium and increase in nutrients such as fibers and vitamins, which is currently voluntary, without compromising the palatability of foods produced. Considering the high intake of milk products as an opportunity to increase other nutrient intake, its quality and composition could be modified to enhance the nutritional content. Fiber, ω-3 fatty acids, and vitamins, which are commonly deficient in this age group, could be introduced to create milk-rich products. Growing-up formulas could be considered, but prices are one of the possible factors to prevent it.

Even with the intention of the food industry to provide adequate milk substitutes during feeding transition, people still choose to feed their toddlers with products based on cow's milk for economic reasons. An initiative may consider public and private subsidies to provide adequate milk substitutes for people who cannot afford it. Governments should control the aggressive marketing of energy-dense and nutrient-poor foods and beverages directed at children. Technologies and new communication spaces as digital influencers can be used to transmit positive messages regarding healthy feeding. Children may use them as models and examples, so they can play an important role in children's eating habits.

Brazilian food diversity should be explored. Why do we see diversity in food production but not in food intake and equal availability? To reduce inequality in food access, a possible initiative could be reducing food wasting, especially during distribution. Creative cooking skills presented in a socially vulnerable community using the variety of fruits and vegetables available in the country are one way to promote healthy eating habits.

A favorable environment for translating intentions to improve children's feeding into practice is essential. This includes an integrated system involving families, schools, governments, and the food industry. With the commitment of all sectors involved in children feeding, effective outcomes could be achieved in order to reduce children's overweight and obesity and promote healthy eating habits that will impact their life course (Fig. 2).

Conflict of Interest Statement

M.F. receives speaker fees and research grants from Abbott, Cereal Partners Worldwide (CPW), Danone Research, Novo Nordisk, and Nutrociencia. He was a member of the ILSI (International Life Sciences Institute) Brazil Board of Directors and the Danone Institute International Board. L.D.B. declares no conflicts of interest.

References

1 Instituto Brasileiro de Geografia e Estatística (IBGE): Pesquisa Nacional por Amostra de Domicílios Contínua: rendimento de todas as fontes: 2018. Rio de Janeiro, IBGE, Coordenação de Trabalho e Rendimento, 2018.
2 Bueno MB, Fisberg RM, Maximino P, et al: Nutritional risk among Brazilian children 2–6 years old: a multicenter study. Nutrition 2013;29:405–410.
3 International Policy Centre for Inclusive Growth. The Food Security Policy Context in Brazil. Country Study. Number 22. Brasília, 2011.
4 Instituto Brasileiro de Geografia e Estatística (IBGE): Pesquisa de Orçamentos Familiares 2008–2009: análise do consumo alimentar pessoal no Brasil. Rio de Janeiro, IBGE, Coordenação de Trabalho e Rendimento, 2011.
5 Martins JM: Universal iron fortification of foods: the view of a hematologist. Rev Bras Hematol Hemoter 2012;34: 459–463.
6 Fisberg M, Del'arco APWT, Previdelli NA, Tosatti AM, Nogueira-de-Almeida CA: Between meal snacks and food habits in preschool Brazilian children: national representative sample survey. Int J Nutrol 2015;8:58-71.
7 Saldiva SRDM, Venancio SI, de Santana AC, et al: The consumption of unhealthy foods by Brazilian children is influenced by their mother's educational level. Nutr J 2014;13:33.
8 Bortolini GA, Vitolo MR, Gubert MB, Santos LMP: Early cow's milk consumption among Brazilian children: results of a national survey. J Pediatr (Rio J) 2013;89:608–613.
9 Maximino P, Machado RHV, Ricci R, et al: Children with feeding difficulties tend to high protein and milk-based supplements' intake – how to break this cycle? Demetra 2019;14:1–17.
10 Haines J, Haycraft E, Lytle L, et al: Nurturing children's healthy eating: position statement. Appetite 2019;137:124–133.

Published online: November 9, 2020

Black MM, Singhal A, Hillman CH (eds): Building Future Health and Well-Being of Thriving Toddlers and Young Children. Nestlé Nutr Inst Workshop Ser. Basel, Karger, 2020, vol 95, pp 33–40 (DOI: 10.1159/000511514)

Growth Faltering: Underweight and Stunting

Andrew M. Prentice

MRC Unit The Gambia at London School of Hygiene and Tropical Medicine, Banjul, Gambia

Abstract

The great majority of attention on growth faltering concentrates on the first "1,000 days" with a much lesser focus on toddlers and young preschoolers. The rationale for this is understandable since the first 1,000 days cover the period of most rapid growth and changes in body composition, the period of breastfeeding, and the complex transition from breastfeeding and weaning to complementary feeds, and then moving to the family/adult diet. There has also been a strong perception that, once a child has become stunted or wasted in the first 2 years of life, there is little hope of recovery, an assumption we address below. This paper will describe the timing of the development of stunting and wasting, addressing 3 critical periods: intergenerational, in utero, and early postnatal life. The question of whether toddlers and young preschoolers can recover from stunting and wasting will also be addressed; our own studies suggest that a degree of recovery is certainly possible. The hormonal mechanisms regulating early growth will be examined. Finally, the issue of whether toddlers and young preschoolers should have special foods and diets will also be discussed.

Introduction

The great majority of attention on growth faltering concentrates on the first "1,000 days" with a much lesser focus on toddlers and young preschoolers. The rationale for this is understandable: the first 1,000 days cover the period of most

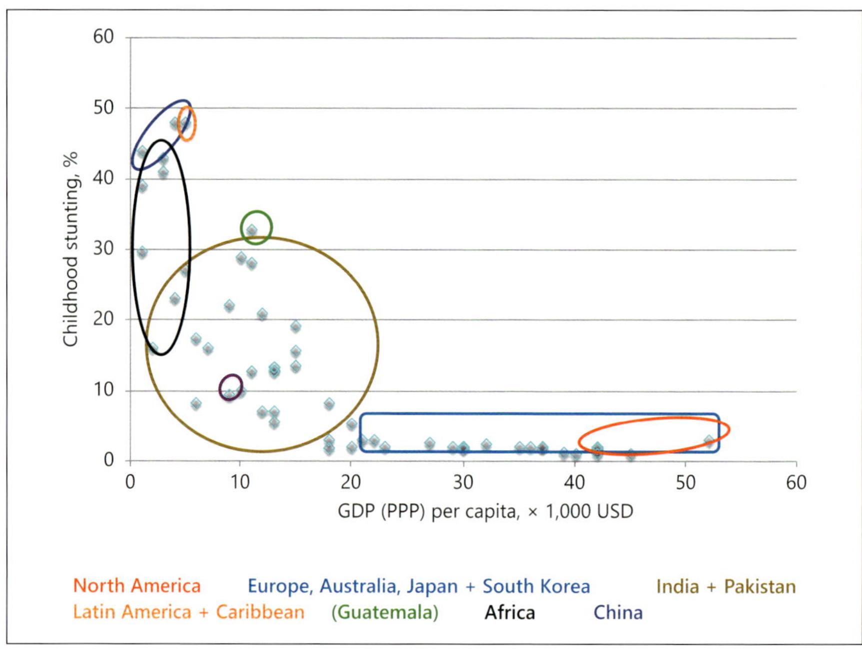

Fig. 1. Childhood stunting is predominantly a problem of low-income countries and resolves rapidly with economic advancement. Data compiled from Demographic Health Surveys since 2005. GDP, gross domestic product; PPP, purchasing power parity.

rapid growth and developmental changes in body composition (especially with respect to brain growth); it is the period of breastfeeding and of the complex transition from breastfeeding as the child is weaned onto complementary feeds; and in the second year of postnatal life, the child starts to adopt the family/adult diet. There has also been a strong perception that once a child has become stunted or wasted in the first 2 years of life, there is little hope of recovery [1] – an assumption we address below.

Global Distribution of Stunting, Wasting, and Underweight in Toddlers and Young Preschoolers

It is self-evident that, with the exception of certain rare clinical conditions or inappropriate parenting behaviors, stunting, wasting, and the consequent underweight are largely confined to the poorer populations of low-income countries. As some of these countries emerge from poverty and pass through the economic transition, malnutrition rates fall sharply and soon resemble those in first-world nations (Fig. 1); a corollary is that obesity rates rise rapidly as will be discussed elsewhere in this symposium [2]. In 2012, the World Health Organization (WHO) estimated that there were 162 million stunted children worldwide and established a "Comprehensive Implementation Plan on Maternal, Infant, and Young Child Nutrition" that set one of the "Global Nutrition Targets" to reduce this number by 40% by the year 2025 [3]. Two-fifths of these children are in the toddler and preschooler age group (defined as 2–5 years for the purposes of this paper), and because there is only limited scope for recovering growth deficits during this period, the greater emphasis on interventions must be placed on earlier periods, as discussed below.

Timing of the Development of Stunting and Wasting

There are 3 critical periods in the development of stunting.

The first of these relates to the generations before a child is even conceived. There is clear evidence for intergenerational influences on population height, and it usually takes a number of generations for these influences to wash out as populations move to conditions of improved diets and living conditions [4]. In this field, there is a subtle but important terminological distinction between *intergenerational* influences and *transgenerational* influences [5]. The former can be mediated through a mother's small body size which can impart effects through numerous possible mechanisms such as "uterine constraints." The evidence for these effects is robust. To take a single example, Young et al. [6] described the relationship between the preconception maternal nutritional status and stunting at 2 years of age in the PRECONCEPT study in Vietnam. A height <150 cm was associated with an incident risk ratio of 1.85 and a weight of <43 kg with a risk of 1.35 for stunting at 2 years [6].

Much less certain is whether there can be transgenerational effects in humans. Such effects would not be mediated by the direct influence of a mother's diet or body size. Transgenerational effects would therefore require some method (e.g., epigenetic programming marks that survive erasure in the very early embryo) that would convey a signal that would affect stunting; we have some evidence that this can occur [7], but much more research is needed.

The second critical period is in utero, and it has been shown that a substantial proportion of childhood stunting and wasting has its origins in fetal life, especially in the last trimester of pregnancy when growth rates are proportionately faster than at any other period of life. A meta-analysis of data from 19 studies in low- and middle-income countries has shown that, relative to appropriate-for-gestational-age and term babies, the risks of stunting in the age range from 12 to 60 months is 1.93 for appropriate-for-gestational-age but preterm babies, 2.43

for small-for-gestational-age and term babies, and 4.51 for small-for-gestational-age and preterm babies [8].

The third critical window is in the early postnatal period. Child growth is under hormonal control, and there are 3 recognized growth stages: fetal, infant, and child (and later adolescence) growth [9]. Fetal growth is largely driven by insulin (produced by the fetal pancreas). Infant growth is driven by insulin and IGF1 independently of growth hormone regulation. Then there is a transition, the so-called infant-to-child transition (ICT), as growth hormone starts to exert its control on the pace of growth; this is the period relevant to toddlers' and young preschoolers' growth, and delayed ICT is a recognized clinical syndrome [10]. Karlberg [9], the original proponent of ICT, hypothesized that poor growth of children in low-income settings may be due to a delayed ICT. In fact, our latest research suggests that, at least in the rural Gambian children whom we study, there is evidence for advanced ICT which may be problematic in prematurely terminating the fetal-infant period of rapid growth [11]. Additional evidence from our own very detailed studies of growth trajectories suggests that the "channels" that will steer later growth are established surprisingly early in postnatal life [Bernstein et al., in preparation].

Can Toddlers and Young Preschoolers Recover from Stunting and Wasting?

In most poor communities from low- and middle-income countries, there is a precipitous drop-off in average height-for-age *Z*-scores compared to the WHO growth reference. This seems to be caused, in large part, by exposure to infections and highly unhygienic living conditions leading to high levels of morbidity that can impair growth through a number of pathways especially involving a persistently damaged gut mucosa [12]. Analysis of aggregate data from many such countries suggests that there is little evidence for a later recovery (see Victora et al. [1]). However, our own decades-long studies of poor rural Gambian children show that they achieve a catchup of almost 1 *Z*-score between 2 and 5 years of age (Fig. 2). There is a remarkable switch from a negative growth trajectory of about –1 height-for-age *Z*-score per year in the first 2 years of life to a positive trajectory of about +0.2 *Z*-scores in the next 3 years. We interpret this as due to the fact that their immune systems have finally developed a resilience against the great majority of the most prevalent infections. We have also emphasized that there can be a second period of catchup in adolescence [13].

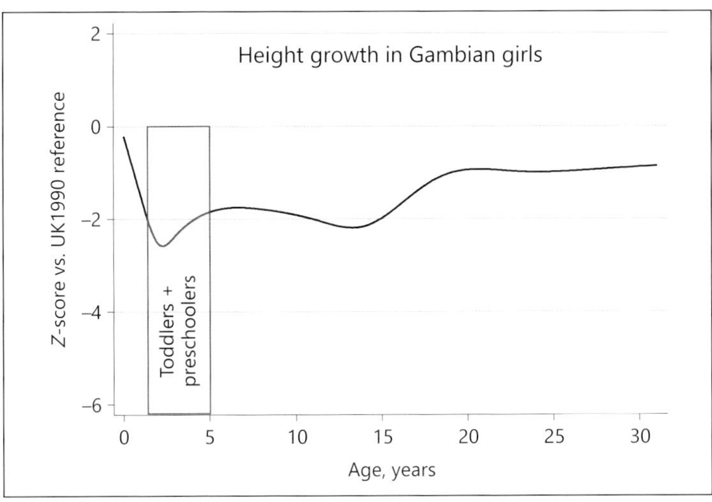

Fig. 2. Toddlers and young preschoolers show slight height catchup following severe faltering in the first 2 years of life (modified from Prentice et al. [13] with permission).

Nutrient Needs of Toddlers and Young Preschoolers

Human toddlers and preschoolers grow very slowly compared to the young of other species; this is an evolved mechanism assumed to have been designed primarily to allow plenty of time for the development, wiring, and training of a large and complex brain [14]. A consequence of this slow growth is that the nutrient requirements for deposition of new tissue are low. In early infancy (0–3 months), babies accrue about 2.5 g protein and 19 g fat per day with an energy cost of around 25 kJ/g [15]. The protein requirements required for this slow growth are low. In the first 6 months of life, a baby is estimated to deposit 0.46 g/kg/day of protein in new tissue growth and have a maintenance need of 0.66 g/kg/day giving a total requirement of 1.12 g/kg/day [16]. By 2 years of age, the estimated need for tissue deposition has fallen to 0.13 g/kg/day and by 4 years of age to just 0.03 g/kg/day giving total estimated protein needs of 0.79 and 0.69 g/kg/day.

In terms of energy, the overall estimated requirements are about 430 kJ/kg/day in the first few months of life. By 2–3 years of age, the estimated energy needs have fallen to about 340 kJ/kg/day, and by 4–5 years they have declined further to about 315 kJ/kg/day. The requirements for basic metabolic needs would be lower but for 2 reasons: (a) due to the costs of ambulation and spontaneous physical activity in naturally active young children and (b) because the brain develops a high requirement for glucose [17].

20 Husseini M, Darboe MK, Moore SE, et al: Thresholds of socio-economic and environmental conditions necessary to escape from childhood malnutrition: a natural experiment in rural Gambia. BMC Med 2018;16:199.
21 Nahar B, Hossain MI, Hamadani JD, et al: Effects of psychosocial stimulation on improving home environment and child-rearing practices: results from a community-based trial among severely malnourished children in Bangladesh. BMC Public Health 2012;12:622.
22 Perkins JM, Kim R, Krishna A, et al: Understanding the association between stunting and child development in low- and middle-income countries: next steps for research and intervention. Soc Sci Med 2017;193:101–109.
23 Walker SP, Wachs TD, Gardner JM, et al; International Child Development Steering Group: Child development: risk factors for adverse outcomes in developing countries. Lancet 2007;369:145–157.
24 Walker SP, Wachs TD, Grantham-McGregor S, et al: Inequality in early childhood: risk and protective factors for early child development. Lancet 2011;378:1325–1338.

Published online: November 6, 2020

Black MM, Singhal A, Hillman CH (eds): Building Future Health and Well-Being of Thriving Toddlers and Young Children. Nestlé Nutr Inst Workshop Ser. Basel, Karger, 2020, vol 95, pp 41–51 (DOI: 10.1159/000511510)

Obesity in Toddlers and Young Children: Causes and Consequences

Atul Singhal

Childhood Nutrition Research Centre, Population, Policy, and Practice Research and Teaching Department, UCL Great Ormond Street Institute of Child Health, London, UK

Abstract

The rapid rise in obesity in toddlers and young children (aged 0–5 years) is a major concern for public health globally. Understanding risk factors for obesity in the early years is therefore fundamental to help guide parents, educators, and health care professionals caring for young children and to develop preventative strategies. Most research has focused on biological risk factors, which can be broadly categorized as genetic predisposition, poor diet (and the behaviors that influence excessive food intake), insufficient physical activity, and the role of developmental factors in early life that influence long-term health. The latter includes establishment of dietary habits and dietary patterns in young (preschool) children and the effect of a high protein intake on the increasing risk of later obesity. Other risk factors particularly relevant to young children include inadequate sleep, high consumption of sugar-sweetened drinks, and large food portions. Understanding the causes of obesity in preschool children is particularly important in view of long-term detrimental consequences of obesity in this age group on the risk of obesity and cardiometabolic disease in adults. The present chapter reviews causes of obesity in preschool children and its consequences for long-term health, focusing particularly on modifiable nutritional risk factors.

Introduction

The huge increase in the prevalence of obesity over the last 40 years in nearly all 200 countries studied is a major challenge for health care systems worldwide [1]. According to the World Health Organization (WHO), in 2016, 39% of adults globally were overweight and 13% obese [2]. Importantly, this problem is not confined to adults and high-income countries [1]. In 2016, for instance, over 41 million children under the age of 5 years were overweight or obese, nearly half of whom lived in Asia [2]. Despite this growing threat to the health of populations, treatments for obesity available are few [3], especially those affordable or suitable for low- and middle-income countries. Once established, obesity is difficult to reverse, and most interventions for obesity are expensive and difficult to implement at large scale, and long-term results are disappointing [3]. Hence, prevention of obesity is critical, particularly in the early years where there may be an opportunity to affect the long-term trajectories of weight gain and to induce sustained effects [4, 5].

Several recent reports have highlighted the importance of preventing obesity in the early years. These include the WHO report on ending childhood obesity [4] and the UK Chief Medical Officer's report: "Time to Solve Childhood Obesity" [5]. Both reports emphasize the critical role of the first few years in establishing good nutritional and physical activity behaviors that can help prevent long-term excessive weight gain. This concept is strongly supported by data showing that, in richer countries at least, most excess weight at adolescence is gained before 5 years of age [6, 7]. The present chapter reviews the possible causes of obesity in young children and its consequences on long-term health, focusing particularly on modifiable nutritional risk factors.

Environmental Risk Factors for Obesity

At the simplest level, obesity results from an imbalance between energy intake and energy expenditure. However, childhood obesity cannot be due to an energy imbalance as result of voluntary lifestyle choices, particularly in preschool children. The factors that predispose to a positive energy balance are complex and include genetic predisposition and exposure to an unhealthy "obesogenic" environment, such as the easy availability and affordability of highly palatable, energy-dense foods [4, 5]. Social determinants of health (the conditions in which people are born, grow, work, and live, such as the physical environment) also have a major impact on childhood obesity by, for example, affecting the availability of takeaway food outlets and areas for outdoor active play [5]. Commercial determinants of health (e.g., food production, marketing, and sale) contribute to the risk of a child becoming overweight. For instance, children respond to TV advertising by consuming more energy-dense snacks and foods [8]. However, most research focuses on the biological determinants of obesity, particularly those affecting modifiable risk factors that influence diet and physical activity, but also those affecting the gut microbiome, sleep, psychological responses, and appetite. Not only do these biological, social, and commercial determinants of health interact to increase the risk of obesity, they also contribute strongly to wide socioeconomic inequalities in this risk. For instance, amongst 4- to 5-year-old children in the UK, obesity in the most deprived 10% of the population is 6% greater than the least deprived decile, a disparity that has been increasing over the last 10 years [5].

Despite the key role of the obesogenic environment, many children living in such an environment do not become obese. Therefore, the risk of becoming overweight is highly variable and depends on a child's biological and behavioral response to the environment. A child's biological response to an obesogenic environment is strongly influenced by genetic factors and by "developmental" or early-life factors that "program" or influence long-term health [9]. The behavioral response of preschool children in particular depends on their parent's behavior, which is in turn strongly influenced by parental socioeconomic status, knowledge, ethnicity, and cultural background. For example, parents may fail to recognize that the child has a weight problem, or behaviors such as eating while watching TV may increase the risk of obesity [10]. A lack of knowledge or social or financial resources may also prevent parents from making healthy food choices [11].

Given the myriad of interacting biological, social, and commercial determinants of obesity, identifying individual causal factors is both complex and challenging. Hence, this review will focus on genetic, dietary, and developmental factors most commonly linked to childhood obesity and most relevant to children under 5 years of age.

Genetic Risk Factors

Children born in families where both parents are obese have a >10-fold greater risk of becoming obese themselves [12]. Although this increased risk could be either due to genetic mechanisms or shared familial characteristics such as diet, twin studies and adoption studies (in which identical twins are raised in different families) suggest that 40–70% of the interindividual variability in body mass index (BMI) is attributable to genetic factors [13]. Relatively few individual genes (e.g., melanocortin 4 receptor, fat mass and obesity-associated [or FTO] gene, leptin, leptin receptor, and the proopiomelanocortin genes) have been identified, many of which lead to severe early-onset obesity by influencing the leptin-melanocortin pathway, a regulator of energy intake [13]. More recently, genome-wide association studies have identified >97 genetic BMI loci, with each locus making a small contribution to the total risk (the strongest being the FTO gene) [13]. Aggregating these individual genetic variants to provide a genetic risk score shows that individuals with a high polygenic risk score (top 10% of the population) have a fourfold greater risk of developing obesity than the bottom 10%, an effect that is evident in preschool children [14]. Interestingly, the genetic contribution to BMI appears to be greater in children than in adults [15].

However, although genes affect an *individual's* risk of becoming overweight, the huge rise in population obesity over the last 40 years is simply too great and too rapid to be explained predominantly by genetic factors [5]. Observations that intraindividual variance in body weight is similar to interindividual variance argue against a tight (genetic) control of body weight [16], and the fact that 97 loci for BMI explain only 2.7% of the variance in population BMI also argues against a dominant role for genetic factors in the risk of childhood obesity [13].

Nutritional Risk Factors

Given their role in energy imbalance, nutritional factors such as energy intake would be expected to be the strongest contributors to obesity in children. However, although diets of preschool children often do not comply with current recommendations [17], there is surprisingly little evidence of an association between diet and risk of obesity, possibly because of limitations in accurately measuring dietary intake in young children [17]. For instance, higher total energy intake is inconsistently associated with obesity (as reviewed [17]), while the macronutrient source of the energy, such as total carbohydrate or fat intake, also does not affect adiposity [17]. In support of this, a Cochrane systematic review found little consistent evidence of an association between fat intake and body fatness in children [18], while a systematic review of 81 studies found inconclusive associations between dietary factors and 12 obesity-related biomarkers (e.g., blood lipids) [19]. In contrast to fat and carbohydrates, protein intake in preschool children may affect *later* (as opposed to current) risk of obesity [20] and is therefore discussed under developmental risk factors below.

Another approach to identifying specific nutritional risk factors for childhood obesity is to consider changes in dietary habits and foods consumed since the onset of the obesity epidemic. Over the last 100 years, overall energy intake has fallen alongside the fall in physical activity, but since the 1970s substantial increases in total energy intake have driven the obesity epidemic and can explain most of the increase in adult body weight (as reviewed [5]). The diets of preschool children in the UK have changed markedly, and today's children have a far greater intake of sugar and soft drinks, and eat less vegetables than those of a similar age in the 1950s (a time of postwar austerity) [21]. Furthermore, concurrent increases in obesity, together with increases in both the size of food portions and dietary energy density, suggest these specific nutritional factors could be particularly important in excessive weight gain in young children.

Sugar and Sugar-Sweetened Beverages

The parallel increases in obesity and sugar consumption (particularly sugar-sweetened beverages, SSBs) suggests a key role for high sugar foods in the development of childhood obesity. Although infants have an innate preference for sweet tastes, there is no nutritional requirement for free sugars (defined as "all monosaccharides/disaccharides added to foods/beverages, plus sugars naturally present in honey/syrups/unsweetened fruit juices and fruit juice concentrates, but not sugar naturally present in intact fruits and lactose naturally present in human and other milks") [22]. Prospective cohort studies and randomized controlled trials (RCTs) have consistently shown that high free sugar intake increases the risk of obesity in children and adults (as summarized in systematic reviews from the WHO, UK Scientific Advisory Committee for Nutrition [SACN], and European Society for Paediatric Gastroenterology, Hepatology, and Nutrition – ESPGHAN [22]). Recent systematic reviews suggest that this association is most consistent in children aged <5 years [23], and that strategies to reduce SSB consumption are effective in this age group [24]. However, few studies have investigated the impact of such interventions on adiposity (probably because of widely recognized difficulties in achieving long-term compliance with dietary interventions). Nonetheless, there is sufficient evidence for public health bodies such as SACN and ESPGHAN to recommend reducing free sugar to less than 5% of daily energy intake in children aged 2–18 years and to even less in those under 2 years [22]. For an average 3-year-old child, this equates to 13 g free sugar/day (<3 teaspoons) or an average of 170 mL of fruit juice/day [22]. In practice, this means consuming sugar as part of a main meal and in a natural form, such as human milk, milk, unsweetened dairy products, and fresh fruits, and replacing fruit juice with water or unsweetened milk drinks. In addition, as recommended by the WHO [4], several countries (e.g., the UK, Mexico, Colombia, Chile, South Africa, and France) have successfully applied taxes to reduce SSB consumption. For instance, in the UK, a levy of 24 p/L on drinks containing >8 g/100 mL of sugar, and 18 p/L on those with 5–8 g/100 mL, has reduced the total sugar content of soft drinks sold before (2015) and after the tax (2018) by 30,100 tons or 21% [5].

Portion Size

Concurrent with the increase in obesity over the last 30 years, there has been a marked increase in the size of food portions given to children [25]. When children and adults are offered larger servings of energy-dense foods, overall energy intake increases (the so-called "portion size effect" [25]). Interestingly, in one of the first studies to show this, energy intake increased in children aged 5 years, but not 3 years, suggesting that younger children have better self-regulation of energy intake [26]. A systematic review of 6 intervention studies has confirmed the portion size effect in 3- to 5-year-old children, particularly in those >4 years [27], consistent with the idea that younger children have better self-regulation of appetite [26]. The effect has been seen most recently in a crossover RCT in 3- to 5-year-old children, which found offering larger portions resulted in higher energy intake (10–15% above calculated needs), with the greatest increases observed in more overweight children [28]. Larger servings (but notably not meal frequencies), were also associated with greater weight gain in twins aged 2–5 years (n = 1,939) [29], supporting the idea that providing practical advice on portion size could help prevent excessive weight gain [25].

Physical Activity, Sedentary Behavior, and Sleep

A lack of physical activity would be expected to contribute to a positive energy balance and hence the risk of obesity. This concept is supported by a systematic review in 0- to 4-year-old children, which reported that physical activity was associated with adiposity in 16 observational studies and 2 RCTs [30]. However, the same review found that 30 studies showed no association between physical activity and adiposity, and 4 even showed an unfavorable effect [30]. Moreover, a meta-analysis (n = 1,100) of 3 cluster RCTs and 1 nonrandomized intervention found no differences in BMI between intervention and control groups. Whilst physical activity has been consistently shown to have many health benefits in preschool children (e.g., for cardiometabolic and psychological health, and physical, motor, and cognitive development [30]), a causal link with obesity has not been established. For instance, a recent Cochrane systematic review found that interventions for obesity prevention that focused on physical activity alone were not effective in children aged 0–5 years [31]. Nonetheless, physical activity is an essential component of a healthy lifestyle, and, in the UK, 3 h of any intensity play (including active and outdoor play) per day is recommended for children aged 1–4 years.

Unsurprisingly, a low level of physical activity is associated with greater sedentary behavior, defined as low-energy sitting or reclining during waking hours [32]. Sedentary behavior, such as the time spent in front of a screen, is postulated to be a risk factor for obesity independent of the time spent in moderate or vigorous physical activity. However, there is little evidence to support this widely accepted hypothesis in young children. For example, a systematic review of 60 studies that included 1 RCT and 13 longitudinal studies found no overall evidence for associations between objectively measured total sedentary time and health indicators (including adiposity) in children aged 0–4 years (as opposed to older children and adults) [32].

A third behavior linked to adiposity in children is inadequate sleep. Two recent systematic reviews have confirmed that insufficient sleep is associated with obesity in preschool children [33, 34]. A meta-analysis of 7 cohorts found that "short" sleepers aged 0–3 years had a 40% (95% CI: 19–65%) greater risk of being overweight or obese >1 year later [34]. The mechanisms are unknown, but a systematic review of 5 studies showed that poor sleep in preschool children was associated with poor diet quality and greater energy intake [35]. Although there is no casual evidence for a link between sleep and obesity, sleep has clearly numerous health benefits for preschool children. However, many young children fail to get enough sleep (e.g., 10–13 h per 24 h for children aged 3–5 years recommended by the American Academy of Pediatrics). Improving sleep may therefore be a worthwhile target for public health interventions [4, 5].

Overall, although more physical activity, less sedentary behavior, and adequate sleep have huge health benefits in their own right, the scientific consensus is that the rise in childhood obesity is mostly driven by changes in food consumption rather than declines in physical activity [5]. Therefore, as recommended by the UK Chief Medical Officer [5], 80% of effort for obesity prevention should focus on improving the diet and 20% on increasing physical activity.

Developmental Factors

There is increasing evidence that developmental factors act in the early years to "program" or influence long-term risk of obesity, a concept known as the developmental origins of health and disease [9, 20]. A systematic review of 282 prospective studies identified consistent associations between several such factors acting in the first 1,000 days (the period between conception and age 2 years) and later obesity, including maternal prepregnancy BMI, prenatal tobacco exposure, maternal excess gestational weight gain, high infant birth weight, and accelerated infant weight gain [9]. Fewer studies also supported a role for gestational diabetes, child care attendance, low strength of maternal-infant relationship, low socioeconomic status, curtailed infant sleep, inappropriate bottle use, introduction to solid food intake before age 4 months, and infant antibiotic exposure [9]. However, most studies are observational, and because of possible confounding, evidence of causality is limited. For instance, associations between gut microbiota (affected by antibiotic use) and obesity may be confounded because both exposure (microbiome) and outcome (obesity) are strongly affected by an unhealthy diet poor in fruit and vegetables.

One developmental factor where there is more causal evidence is the impact of accelerated growth in infancy (usually as a result of higher protein intake) on later obesity. This hypothesis is supported by several RCTs [36] and seems to include effects of accelerated growth/higher protein intake in toddlers. For instance, a systematic review of 13 studies found that a higher protein intake between 6 and 36 months was associated with higher BMI later in childhood (pooled effect size 0.28 BMI *Z*-scores; 95% CI: 0.20–0.35) [17, 37]. The mechanisms for these effects are unknown but may involve programming of IGF-1 concentrations or effects on appetite regulation [36]. Since cow's milk is the major source of protein in young children, limiting cow's milk intake has been suggested as a possible intervention for obesity prevention (e.g., by ESPGHAN) [36].

Another development factor particularly related to obesity in toddlers is programming of dietary habits and food preferences that can influence lifelong health. Analysis of children's diets by deriving a limited number of dietary patterns from a large variety of foods eaten using principal component analysis strongly supports this concept. These dietary patterns emerge in early life, are established by 3 years of age, and are stable (or track) throughout childhood and into adult life (as reviewed [17]). As expected, unhealthy dietary patterns in children including toddlers are associated with a greater risk of later obesity [38]. However, in the absence of intervention studies, the question of whether the diets of young children can be manipulated to ameliorate this risk is not known.

Consequences of Childhood Obesity

Many cohort studies, and more recently mendelian randomization studies, have established clear causal links between obesity in adults and adverse health consequences such cardiovascular disease, type 2 diabetes, and cancer [13]. However, although the detrimental effects of obesity in older children and adults are well recognized, health care professionals and parents often fail to appreciate its harmful effects in toddlers and preschool children. Nevertheless, there is strong evidence for adverse consequences of excess weight in toddlers on both short- and long-term health.

In the immediate or short term, obesity in children is associated with problems resembling those in adults, such as sleep apnea, asthma, back and joint pain, and components of the metabolic syndrome such as high-blood pressure, raised cholesterol, fatty liver disease, and increased risk of type 2 diabetes [5]. In fact, in the UK, there are 100 new cases of type 2 diabetes diagnosed in children each year [5]. Some complications of obesity are unique to children such as slipped femoral epiphyses and premature puberty [5]. Other immediate complications of obesity may be more marked in children, such as psychological consequences, poor cognitive function and brain health, depression, and bullying leading to low self-esteem and poor educational attainment [5]. All of these comorbidities have a major impact on the individual, parents, and health care services. However, of particular public health concern are the long-term consequences of childhood obesity on *adult* health. Obese children are 5 times more likely to become obese adults [5], and several systematic reviews have shown associations between obesity in preschool children (0–6 years) and the metabolic syndrome in adults [39] and between obesity in older children (>7 years) and adult type 2 diabetes, cardiovascular disease, and cancer [40]. Alarmingly, these effects seem to persist even in obese children who become slim adults.

Overview

Understanding the reasons behind the rapid increase in obesity in toddlers and young children over the last 50 years is a major challenge for scientists, health care professionals, and policy makers worldwide. Although causality is often difficult to establish, many risk factors have been identified which act at both a societal and individual level. However, childhood obesity is complex and multifactorial, with each factor likely to make only a small contribution to the overall risk. Interventions for obesity prevention therefore need to target multiple risk factors and be implemented at society, community, and family level. Nonetheless, there is little doubt that investing in obesity prevention in the early years will have huge health and economic benefits for populations, children, and the wider society [5].

Conflict of Interest Statement

The author declares no conflict of interest.

References

1 NCD Risk Factor Collaboration (NCD-RisC): Worldwide trends in body-mass index, underweight, overweight, and obesity from 1975 to 2016: a pooled analysis of 2,416 population-based measurement studies in 128·9 million children, adolescents, and adults. Lancet 2017;390:2627–2642.

2 World Health Organization: Obesity and Overweight Fact Sheet. Geneva, WHO, 2018. https://www.who.int/en/news-room/fact-sheets/detail/obesity-and-overweight.

3 Heymsfield SB, Wadden TA: Mechanisms, pathophysiology, and management of obesity. N Engl J Med 2017;376:254–266.

4 World Health Organization: Report of the Commission on Ending Childhood Obesity. Geneva, WHO, 2016. https://www.who.int/end-childhood-obesity/publications/echo-report/en/.

5 Davies SC: Time to Solve Childhood Obesity, Department of Health Social Care 2019. https://www.gov.uk/government/organisations/department-of-health-and-social-care.

6 Gardner DS, Hosking J, Metcalf BS, et al: Contribution of early weight gain to childhood overweight and metabolic health: a longitudinal study (EarlyBird 36). Pediatrics 2009;123:e67–e73.

7 Geserick M, Vogel M, Gausche R, et al: Acceleration of BMI in early childhood and risk of sustained obesity. N Engl J Med 2018;379:1303–1312.

8 Norman J, Kelly B, McMahon AT, et al: Sustained impact of energy-dense TV and online food advertising on children's dietary intake: a within-subject, randomised, crossover, counter-balanced trial. Int J Behav Nutr Phys Act 2018;15:37.

9 Woo Baidal JA, Locks LM, Cheng ER, et al: Risk factors for childhood obesity in the first 1,000 days: a systematic review. Am J Prev Med 2016;50:761–779.

10 Ghobadi S, Hassanzadeh-Rostami Z, Salehi-Marzijarani M, et al: Association of eating while television viewing and overweight/obesity among children and adolescents: a systematic review and meta-analysis of observational studies. Obes Rev 2018;19:313–320.

11 Mazarello Paes V, Ong KK, Lakshman R: Factors influencing obesogenic dietary intake in young children (0–6 years): systematic review of qualitative evidence. BMJ Open 2015;5:e007396.

12 Reilly JJ, Armstrong J, Dorosty AR, et al: Early life risk factors for obesity in childhood: cohort study. BMJ 2005;330:1357.

13 Goodarzi MO: Genetics of obesity: what genetic association studies have taught us about the biology of obesity and its complications. Lancet Diabetes Endocrinol 2018;6:223–236.

14 Khera AV, Chaffin M, Wade KH, et al: Polygenic prediction of weight and obesity trajectories from birth to adulthood. Cell 2019;177:587–596.e9.

15 Elks CE, den Hoed M, Zhao JH, et al: Variability in the heritability of body mass index: a systematic review and meta-regression. Front Endocrinol (Lausanne) 2012;3:29.

16 Müller MJ, Geisler, C, Blundell J, et al: The case of GWAS of obesity: does body weight control play by the rules? Int J Obes (Lond) 2018;42:1395–1405.

17 Lanigan J: Prevention of overweight and obesity in early life. Proc Nutr Soc 2018;77:247–256.

18 Naude CE, Visser ME, Nguyen KA, et al: Effects of total fat intake on bodyweight in children. Cochrane Database Syst Rev 2018;7:CD012960.

19 Hilger-Kolb J, Bosle C, Motoc I, et al: Associations between dietary factors and obesity-related biomarkers in healthy children and adolescents – a systematic review. Nutr J 2017;16:85.

20 Patro-Gołąb B, Zalewski BM, Kołodziej M, et al: Nutritional interventions or exposures in infants and children aged up to 3 years and their effects on subsequent risk of overweight, obesity and body fat: a systematic review of systematic reviews. Obes Rev 2016;17:1245–1257.

21 Prynne CJ, Paul AA, Price GM, et al: Food and nutrient intake of a national sample of 4-year-old children in 1950: comparison with the 1990s. Public Health Nutr 1999;2:537–547.

22 Fidler Mis N, Braegger C, Bronsky J, et al: ESPGHAN Committee on Nutrition: Sugar in infants, children and adolescents: a position paper of the European Society for Paediatric Gastroenterology, Hepatology and Nutrition Committee on Nutrition. J Pediatr Gastroenterol Nutr 2017;65:681–696.

23 Frantsve-Hawley J, Bader JD, Welsh JA, et al: A systematic review of the association between consumption of sugar-containing beverages and excess weight gain among children under age 12. J Public Health Dent 2017;77(suppl 1):S43–S66.

24 Vercammen KA, Frelier JM, Lowery CM, et al: A systematic review of strategies to reduce sugar-sweetened beverage consumption among 0-year to 5-year olds. Obes Rev 2018;19:1504–1524.

25 Hetherington MM, Blundell-Birtill P, Caton SJ, et al: Understanding the science of portion control and the art of downsizing. Proc Nutr Soc 2018;77:347–355.

26 Rolls BJ, Engell D, Birch LL: Serving portion size influences 5-year-old but not 3-year-old children's food intakes. J Am Diet Assoc 2000;100:232–234.

27 Small L, Lane H, Vaughan L, et al: A systematic review of the evidence: the effects of portion size manipulation with children and portion education/training interventions on dietary intake with adults. Worldviews Evid Based Nurs 2013;10:69–81.
28 Smethers AD, Roe LS, Sanchez CE, et al: Portion size has sustained effects over 5 days in preschool children: a randomized trial. Am J Clin Nutr 2019;109:1361–1372.
29 Syrad H, Llewellyn CH, Johnson L, et al: Meal size is a critical driver of weight gain in early childhood. Sci Rep 2016;6:28368.
30 Carson V, Lee EY, Hewitt L, et al: Systematic review of the relationships between physical activity and health indicators in the early years (0–4 years). BMC Public Health 2017;17(suppl 5):854.
31 Brown T, Moore TH, Hooper L, et al: Interventions for preventing obesity in children. Cochrane Database Syst Rev 2019;7:CD001871.
32 Poitras VJ, Gray CE, Janssen X, et al: Systematic review of the relationships between sedentary behaviour and health indicators in the early years (0–4 years). BMC Public Health 2017;17(suppl 5):868.
33 Chaput JP, Gray CE, Poitras VJ, et al: Systematic review of the relationships between sleep duration and health indicators in the early years (0–4 years). BMC Public Health 2017;17(suppl 5): 855.
34 Miller MA, Kruisbrink M, Wallace J, et al: Sleep duration and incidence of obesity in infants, children, and adolescents: a systematic review and meta-analysis of prospective studies. Sleep 2018;41.
35 Ward AL, Reynolds AN, Kuroko S, et al: Bidirectional associations between sleep and dietary intake in 0–5 year old children: a systematic review with evidence mapping. Sleep Med Rev 2019;49:101231.
36 Singhal A: The role of infant nutrition in the global epidemic of non-communicable disease. Proc Nutr Soc 2016;75:162–168.
37 Lanigan J, Adegboye A, Northstone K, et al: Nutrition in preschool children and later risk of obesity: a systematic review and meta-analysis. J Pediatr Gastroenterol Nutr 2017;62(suppl 1):691.
38 Liberali R, Kupek E, de Assis MAA: Dietary patterns and childhood obesity risk: a systematic review. Child Obes 2020;16:70–85.
39 Kim J, Lee I, Lim S: Overweight or obesity in children aged 0 to 6 and the risk of adult metabolic syndrome: a systematic review and meta-analysis. J Clin Nurs 2017;26:3869–3880.
40 Llewellyn A, Simmonds M, Owen CG, et al: Childhood obesity as a predictor of morbidity in adulthood: a systematic review and meta-analysis. Obes Rev 2016;17:56–67.

Published online: November 9, 2020

Black MM, Singhal A, Hillman CH (eds): Building Future Health and Well-Being of Thriving Toddlers and Young Children. Nestlé Nutr Inst Workshop Ser. Basel, Karger, 2020, vol 95, pp 52–53 (DOI: 10.1159/000511522)

Summary on Challenges in Nutrition in Toddlers and Young Children

Toddlerhood, the period between 12 and 36 months of age, is a particularly rapid period of human development when new skills such as walking, talking, eating, and bowel and bladder control are mastered. Along with enhanced cognition and social development, these skills enable a child to explore their environment, express themselves, and develop more independence such as self-feeding. However, increasing autonomy, together with behaviors such as impulsivity and food neophobia (defined as refusal or fear of eating unfamiliar foods, a normal developmental phase during toddlerhood), can make mealtimes particularly challenging. Parental feeding practices such as providing opportunities for toddlers to eat healthy foods in age-appropriate settings and responding to a toddler's signals promptly, appropriately, and with nurturance (a pattern known as responsive feeding) are therefore essential for the development of healthy feeding behaviors.

Rapid growth and development in toddlers, in turn, leads to changing nutritional needs. To meet these needs, toddlers need an adequate and varied diet, but few studies have assessed diets of children <5 years of age. Two studies, the South East Asian Nutrition Survey (SEANUTS), conducted in Indonesia, Malaysia, Thailand, and Vietnam, and the Feeding Infants and Toddlers Study (FITS) in the USA have helped identify suboptimal diets in toddlers. Globally, deficiencies in iron, zinc, vitamin A, and iodine are common, and intakes of dietary fiber and vitamin D are generally below recommended levels. These nutritional gaps have consequences on the health of young children in low-, middle-, and high-income countries.

In low-income countries, a common consequence of suboptimal nutrition is stunting, a problem affecting 162 million children globally in 2012 (40% of whom were children aged 2–5 years). This growth faltering occurs predominantly in the first 1,000 days (the period from conception to age 2 years) and often shows little recovery after 2 years of age. However, stunting is not caused by poor diet alone. For example, Gambian children show some catch-up growth between 2 and 5 years of age, possibly as a consequence of fewer infections as their immune systems mature in toddlerhood. Toddlers in low-income countries generally share the adult diet and eat from the family bowl, and so they have limited access to a nutrient-enriched diet to support rapid growth. However, this also means they have lower exposure to "junk" foods.

In middle-income countries, problems of nutritional excess and "hidden hunger" often co-exist in young children. In Brazil for example, 30% of children have excess weight, but micronutrient deficiencies such as iron and vitamin A deficiencies are common in both undernourished and overweight children. Brazilian toddlers have nutritionally poor diets with low intakes of meat, fruits, and vegetables, and high intakes of fried foods, soft drinks, salty snacks, sweets, and cow's milk. Improving toddler diets is therefore essential but needs to go beyond promoting nutritional education and has to involve families, schools, governments, and the food industry.

In high-income countries, obesity is the most important nutritional issue facing toddlers. Causes of obesity in this age group are complex and include social, commercial, and biological determinants of health. Biological risk factors include genetic predisposition, poor diet (and the behaviors that influence excessive food intake), physical inactivity, and the role of developmental factors in early life that influence long-term health (e.g., the impact of a high-protein intake in increasing later risk of obesity). Other risk factors particularly relevant to young children include inadequate sleep, high consumption of sugar-sweetened drinks, and large food portions. Obesity in toddlers has adverse consequences on their short-term health, but also increases the risk of obesity and cardiometabolic diseases in later life. Optimizing nutrition in toddlers is therefore a critical public health priority worldwide.

Atul Singhal

Published online: November 9, 2020

Black MM, Singhal A, Hillman CH (eds): Building Future Health and Well-Being of Thriving Toddlers and Young Children. Nestlé Nutr Inst Workshop Ser. Basel, Karger, 2020, vol 95, pp 54–66 (DOI: 10.1159/000511517)

Transition from Breastfeeding and Complementary Feeding to Toddler Nutrition in Child Care Settings

Lorrene D. Ritchie[a] Danielle L. Lee[a] Elyse Homel Vitale[b] Lauren E. Au[c]

[a]Division of Agriculture and Natural Resources, Nutrition Policy Institute, University of California, Berkeley, CA, USA; [b]Strategy and Operations, Child Care Food Program Roundtable, Los Angeles, CA, USA; [c]Department of Nutrition, University of California, Davis, CA, USA

Abstract

Child care has broad reach to young children. Yet, not all child care settings have nutrition standards for what and how foods and beverages should be served to infants as they transition to toddlerhood. The purpose of this paper is to describe the development of nutrition recommendations to guide feeding young children in licensed child care settings in the USA, a process that could be adapted in other countries. Nutrition standards were designed by nutrition and child care experts to address *what* and *how* to feed young children, also including the transition from infants to toddlers. Nutrition standards are important for health and can be feasibly implemented in child care settings. Feasibility considerations focused on family child care homes, which typically have fewer resources than child care centers or preschools. Infant standards include recommendations for vegetables, fruits, proteins, grains, and breast milk and other beverages. Also included are recommendations for supporting breastfeeding, introducing complementary foods, and promoting self-regulation in response to hunger and satiety. Toddler standards are expanded to address the frequency as well as types of food groups, and recommendations on beverages, sugar, sodium, and fat. Feeding practice recommendations include meal and snack frequency and style, as well as the promotion of self-regulation among older children.

Importance of the Infant to Toddler Transition

Obesity among US children 2–5 years old has nearly tripled from 5% in 1976 to 14% in 2016 [1]. Dietary risk factors for obesity begin in infancy when energy intakes begin to exceed recommendations [2]. Although rates of breastfeeding have improved in recent years [3], most infants in the USA are bottle fed at some point in the first year of life, and 10–20% are introduced to complementary foods prior to the recommended 4–6 months of age [2–4]. As infants transition into toddlers, dietary patterns worsen and are characterized by inadequate intake of fruits, vegetables, and whole grains, and excessive consumption of sugar-sweetened foods and beverages [5]. For example, in a 2008 study, 16–27% of infants 9–12 months old transitioning into toddlers up to 23 months of age did not consume any fruit on a given day. In contrast, intake of sweetened foods tends to increase rapidly as an infant transitions into toddlerhood resulting in as many or more children consuming a sweetened food than a fruit or vegetable on a given day by the second year of life [2, 6]. By the end of toddlerhood, dietary intakes tend to be established, becoming habits that track into later life [2]. Despite the importance of early life for subsequent nutrition and health, the evidence-based recommendations for the nation, the Dietary Guidelines for Americans, do not currently include guidance for young children 0–2 years of age [7].

Role of Child Care in Infant and Toddler Nutrition

Given that over 1 in 5 US children are already overweight or obese before entering kindergarten [1], interventions in the youngest children are essential. Licensed early care and education settings (hereafter referred to as child care) are the largest institutional settings in the USA for improving nutrition among young children. Since the 1970s, the rate of employment by mothers of children under 3 years old has nearly doubled [8]. In 2018, among families with children 0–5 years old, both parents were employed in 58% of households of married couples, and 69% of mothers and 85% of fathers were employed in single-parent households [9]. Concurrent with rates of parent employment, use of child care has risen. Over one-third of all young children spend time in organized, licensed child care (as opposed to informal care with family, friends, or neighbors) [10]. Many young children attend child care for a long day that matches their parent's employment, where they consume much of their daily nutrition [11].

Studies have found mixed associations between attending child care and child obesity [12–14]. For example, in a systematic review of observational studies conducted in developed countries, 3 studies found center-based care associated with increased prevalence of child overweight or obesity, 8 studies found no association, and 2 studies found a protective relationship [12]. Enrollment in full-day child care at an early age (<3 months) has been associated with less breastfeeding and early introduction of complementary foods [15]. Disparities in findings may be partially explained by the timing of exposure to child care. Studies suggest that more time spent in child care, especially during the transition from infancy to toddlerhood in the first and second years of life, is a risk factor for child obesity [13, 14].

In the USA, the federal Child and Adult Care Food Program (CACFP) provides reimbursements to child care centers and homes for up to a total of 3 meals and snacks per day to provide specific types and amounts of food groups [16]. However, relatively few licensed child care facilities participate in this program. In California, for example, which accounts for one-seventh of the US population, only about one-third of young children in licensed child care were at facilities that participate in CACFP [17]. Further, CACFP standards do not regulate foods or beverages that are not claimed for reimbursement and do not specify how children should be fed (e.g., feeding practices). Outside of CACFP, there are no federal nutrition requirements and incomplete and inconsistent state-by-state nutrition requirements to which licensed child care facilities are subject [18]. Few states, for example, have comprehensive standards to support breastfeeding and other recommended early feeding practices in child care [19, 20].

In the USA, licensed facilities can vary from small, family child care homes with a single provider and a few children to large centers or preschools with a director, multiple teachers, and several hundred children. There is concern that nutrition standards may be difficult to afford or implement, particularly by child care homes [21]. Child care homes are independently operated businesses in the homes of providers who often are low-income women with limited resources and opportunities to obtain nutrition training [22]. Further, nutrition in family child care homes tends to be less optimal than in centers or preschools [23].

Developing nutrition standards that are both evidence-based and feasible for implementation in child care settings is an important early step towards laying the groundwork for improving the nutrition of young children. As such, the purpose of this paper is to describe a process whereby evidence-based nutrition standards for young children in child care were developed and refined so that they would be actionable and achievable in most child care settings in the USA, including family child care homes. This process may be adapted to establish or refine nutrition standards for child care settings in other countries.

Development of Child Care Nutrition Standards for Infants and Toddlers

Starting with current guidelines from authoritative bodies, in 2015 standards were refined by both nutrition experts and child care practice-based stakeholders. Science advisors (Table 1) from across the country were selected based on their scientific expertise in nutrition and obesity prevention for children and in child care. They were tasked with developing a comprehensive set of evidence-based nutrition recommendations for: (1) infants from birth up to 1 year of age, and (2) children over 1 year. Science advisors were asked not to include practical considerations of child care settings in their deliberations but focus on standards optimal for child health.

Child care recommendations were first selected from authoritative bodies that had put forward nutrition recommendations for child care settings. These included the CACFP standards [16]; Academy of Nutrition and Dietetics [24]; Nutrition and Physical Activity Self-Assessment for Child Care Best Practices [25]; Institute of Medicine [26]; 2015 Dietary Guidelines for Americans [7]; American Academy of Pediatrics, American Public Health Association and National Resource Center for Health and Safety in Child Care and Early Education's Caring for Our Children [27]; and Nemours [28]. Recommendations on *what* foods and beverages should be offered (dietary intake) as well as *how* the recommended foods and beverages should be offered (feeding practices) were compiled.

The recommendations were tabulated from each expert body and organized by dietary intake of food group (e.g., fruit juice, other fruit, or vegetable) and feeding practices (e.g., breastfeeding or meal service). There were 25 infant nutrition recommendations and 173 child nutrition recommendations identified. To help expedite the process, the most comprehensive nutrition recommendations for each food group or feeding practice were selected prior to the expert convening. Using a Delphi process, group consensus was reached among the science advisors by discussing each highlighted standard and identifying additions, deletions, or revisions. After the completion of this group consensus process, each science advisor independently ranked the nutrition standards according to potential impact (high, medium, and low) on child nutrition, obesity, and health. The science advisor rankings were compiled, and the standards separated into 3 groups according to the following criteria:

- High impact: 70% or more of science advisors ranked as high impact and no science advisor ranked as low impact
- Medium impact: mixed responses from science advisors in between high and low
- Low impact: over 30% of science advisors ranked as low impact, and no science advisor ranked as high impact, or over 50% ranked as low impact.

Table 1. Science advisors involved in the development of infant and toddler nutrition standards child care

Name	Title and affiliation (as of 2015)	Expertise
Karen Cullen, DrPH	Professor, Pediatrics-Nutrition, Baylor College of Medicine	Maternal and child nutrition, W
Jane Heinig, PhD	Academic Administrator, Department of Nutrition Director and International Board-Certified Lactation Consultant, Human Lactation Center, University of California, Davis	Maternal and child nutrition
Kathryn Henderson, PhD	Independent Consultant (formerly Director of School and Community Initiatives and Associate Scientist at the Rudd Center for Food Policy and Obesity at Yale University)	Child obesity prevention
Donna Johnson, PhD	Professor, Health Services, University of Washington	Public health nutrition, child obesity prevention
Susie Nanney, PhD, MPH, RD	Associate Professor, Department of Family Medicine, and Community Health, University of Minneapolis	Obesity prevention in community settings, health disparities, nutrition policy
Sara Benjamin Neelon, PhD, MPH, RD	Associate Professor, Health Behavior and Society, John Hopkins University	Child nutrition, child care nutrition
Lorrene Ritchie, PhD, RD	Director, Nutrition Policy Institute, and Cooperative Extension Specialist, Division of Agriculture and Natural Resources, University of California	Child nutrition, child obesity prevention, federal nutrition assistance programs
Angela Odoms-Young, PhD	Associate Professor, Kinesiology and Nutrition University of Illinois at Chicago	Child obesity prevention, community-based participatory research, health equity
Dianne Stanton Ward, EdD	Professor, Nutrition, University of North Carolina at Chapel Hill	Child obesity prevention, child care nutrition
Mary Story, PhD, RD	Professor, Community and Family Medicine, and Global Health Associate Director for Academic Programs, Duke University	Child nutrition, child obesity prevention
Elsie Taveras, MD, MPH	Chief, Division of General Academic Pediatrics, Department of Pediatrics, Director, Pediatric Population Health Management, Mass General Hospital for Children Associate Professor of Pediatrics, Harvard Medical School Associate Professor of Nutrition, Harvard School of Public Health	Child obesity prevention and treatment
Shannon E. Whaley, PhD	Director of Research and Evaluation, Public Health Foundation Enterprises-WIC	Child development and nutrition, Special Supplemental Nutrition Assistance Program fo WIC

WIC, Women, Infants and Children.

The next step involved convening an independent group of child care community advisors to review the final set of nutrition standards compiled by the science advisors. The child care community advisors included representation from child care advocates, CACFP sponsoring agencies (who provide training and technical assistance to child care centers and homes participating in CACFP), and family child care provider representatives (unions, resources, and referral networks) (Table 2). The primary goal of this group was to come to a consensus about which of the nutrition standards could be applied without jeopardizing the solvency and operation of licensed child care facilities, namely family child care homes. The group deliberated collectively and then independently rated each standard for ease of implementation (easy, medium, or difficult) taking into account the typical needs and resources of child care settings. The child care community advisor rankings were grouped as follows:

- *difficult*: 70% or more of the child care community advisors ranked as difficult and no child care community advisors ranked as easy;
- *medium*: mixed responses from child care community advisors in between high and low; and
- *easy*: over 30% of child care community advisors ranked as easy and no child care community advisors ranked as difficult, or over 50% ranked as easy.

The nutrition standards were then grouped into tiers based on both impact and feasibility of implementation: tier 1 (easy/high, easy/medium, or medium/high); tier 2 (all other rankings). The tiers were included to provide implementation options to be evaluated by researchers as well as for those that implement programs for child care providers and for policy makers.

The final development step was to pilot test the nutrition standards in 2017 with a sample of 30 licensed family child care providers in the USA (specifically in the state of California) over a 3-month period to assess adherence and challenges in implementation. Providers were given a 2-h in-person training and written information on the standards, and they were asked to select a minimum of 3–5 standards to meet over the next 3 months. Adherence to each standard was assessed by survey and observation at baseline and the 3-month follow-up, and compared over time using paired *t* tests. Among the 12 family child care providers caring for infants, adherence increased from 41 to 59% ($p < 0.01$) for tier 1 infant standards and from 32 to 42% ($p < 0.05$) for infant feeding practice standards (both tiers combined). Changes in tier 2 (32 vs. 29%), food and beverage (49 vs. 63%), and all combined (36 vs. 44%) infant standards were not significant. Among the 30 family child care providers caring for toddlers, adherence increased from 58 to 69% ($p < 0.001$) for tier 2 standards, from 62 to 74% ($p < 0.001$) for food and beverage standards, from 51 to 60% ($p < 0.001$) for feeding practice standards, and from 59 to 68% ($p < 0.001$) for all child standards

Table 2. Child care community advisors involved in the development of infant and toddler nutriti standards for child care

Name	Organization (as of 2015)	Position (as of 2015)
Shanice Boyette	California Department of Social Services, Child Care Licensing Program	Child Care Program Licensin
Aaron Ross	California Department of Social Services, Child Care Licensing Program	Child Care Program Licensin
Kelley Knapp	California Department of Education, Nutrition Services Division	Nutrition Education Consultant
Nina Buthee	California Child Development Administrators Association	Executive Director
Domenica Benitez	California Child Care Resource and Referral Network	Provider Services Manager
Barbara Terrell	California Association for Family Child Care	President
Kula Koenig	American Heart Association	Government Relations
Kate Miller	Children Now	Senior Associate, Early Childhood Policy
Jacqueline Deader	FRAMAX/Child Care Food Program Roundtable	Administrative Director
Debbie Zaragoza	Child Development Associates, Inc./ Child Care Food Program Roundtable	Nutrition Program Manager
Karen Farley	California WIC Association	Executive Director
Tonia McMillian	Family Child Care Provider	Family Child Care Provider
Roseanne Galli-Adams	Family Child Care Provider	Family Child Care Provider
Nanette Rincon-Ksido	Service Employees International Union (SEIU)	External Organizing Director, SEIU Local 99
Bobbie Rose	UCSF School of Nursing, CCHP	BSN, Child Care Consultant
Paula James	Contra Costa Child Care Council, Child Health and Nutrition Program	Director, Child Health and Nutrition Program
Veronica Klinger	YMCA San Diego	Field Services
Natalie Dunaway	California Department of Social Services, Child Care Licensing Program	Child Care Advocate-Norther California
Doris Fredericks	Healthy Living: Nutrition, Fitness, and Mindful Eating	Consultant

CCHP, California Childcare Health Program.

ble 3. Child care nutrition standards for infants (0–12 months)

at foods should be served	
jetables	Offer pureed, mashed, or whole vegetables for infants 6–12 months Vegetables can be fresh, frozen, or canned (all with no added salt, fat, or sugar) for infants 6–12 months Offer dark green, orange, red, or deep yellow vegetables ≥ 1 time per day Do not serve deep-fried or prefried baked vegetables
its	Offer unsweetened whole, mashed, or pureed fruits for infants 6–12 months Fruit can be fresh, frozen, or canned (all with no added sugars) for infants 6–12 months
teins	Offer proteins such as soft cooked egg, beans, meat, poultry, and fish without bones for infants 6–12 months Serve protein foods with no added salt for infants 6–12 months Offer natural cheese ≤1–2 times per day; do not serve cheese food/spread for infants 6–12 months Offer yogurt ≤1 time per day, must have <23 g sugar per 6 oz for infants 6–12 months Do not serve processed meats or deep-fried or prefried meats, poultry, or fish
ains	Offer iron-fortified infant cereals for infants 6–12 months Serve whole grains only Do not serve refined (non-whole) grains or grain-based desserts
ast milk and ier beverages	Support and encourage breastfeeding Offer only breast milk and/or iron-fortified infant formula (as beverage besides water) While breast milk and formula are the best sources of water, begin using a cup for additional drinking water at 6–9 months No other milk (e.g., cow's or soy milk) unless a doctor's note Do not serve 100% juice, juice drinks, or any other beverages
jar, sodium, d fat	Do not serve foods with added sugar or sugar equivalents listed as the first or second ingredient Do not offer foods having a combination of 3 or more kinds of sugar or sugar equivalents Do not serve low-calorie sweeteners or items containing low-calorie sweeteners like diet foods or diet beverages Never offer honey to infants Do not serve high-salt foods (>200 mg sodium per snack item or >480 mg sodium per entrée) Do not add salt at the table Use only liquid nontropical vegetable oils instead of solid fats
w foods should be served	
ttle feeding	Provide adequate refrigerator/storage space for breast milk Hold infant in one's arms or sitting up in one's lap while bottle feeding Never prop bottles; do not allow infants to carry, sleep, or rest with bottle Do not serve solid food and any beverages other than breast milk and iron-fortified infant formula in bottle
roducing id foods	At about 6 months, introduce developmentally appropriate solid foods in age-appropriate portion sizes; only feed solid foods that have been previously introduced, with no problems, by the infant's caregivers Start with iron-fortified infant cereals or pureed meats, then pureed vegetables and fruits, and then other protein-rich foods Introduce foods gradually, one at a time, and wait for at least 3–5 days, watch for allergic reactions such as diarrhea, rash, or vomiting At 9 months, begin self-feeding with finger foods then transition to foods served at the table as developmentally appropriate Encourage older infants to self-feed with their fingers and drink from a cup with assistance Offer solid foods at regular meal and snack times for infants 6–12 months Avoid choking hazards (e.g., by cutting grapes into smaller pieces)

Table 3 (continued)

Self-regulation	Feed younger infants on demand by recognizing feeding cues (e.g., rooting and sucking) Ensure that infants are guided by own feelings of hunger and satiety and are not pressured to eat all that is offered
Meal and snack times	Minimize distractions at mealtime (e.g., no TV, toys, phones, or video games) Use dishware and utensils that are sized appropriately Allow enough time to eat Offer a variety of culturally relevant items When food is provided at celebrations or fundraisers offer only healthy items, such as fruit, vegetables, and water Provider models healthy eating and does not consume other items in front of children At least one child care provider sits with infants at a table and eats the same meals and snacks Include older infants at family style meals where provider and children eat together

combined. Change in tier 1 child standards (60 vs. 67%) was not significant. Slightly over one-third (39%) of providers rated tier 1 infant standards as difficult to implement; 19% of providers rated the tier 1 child standards as difficult to implement. Results of the pilot test suggested that nutrition standards are well accepted and can be feasibly implemented by child care providers.

The final nutrition standards include not only *what* foods and beverages to serve but also *how* to feed infants (Table 3) and toddlers (Table 4). Because few differences were detected in implementation in the pilot intervention between the tiers, it was also concluded that tiers were not necessary. Infant standards include recommendations for vegetables, fruits, proteins, grains, and breast milk and other beverages. Also included are recommendations for bottle feeding, introducing complementary foods, and promoting self-regulation in response to hunger and satiety. Toddler standards are expanded to address the frequency as well as types of food groups and beverages, and include guidance on sugar, sodium, and fat. Feeding practices for toddlers include meal and snack frequency, feeding style, and how to promote self-regulation of intake.

Implications for Research and Practice

Past studies have shown that child care-based interventions, while having mixed results, have shown promising impacts on child dietary intakes [29, 30]. Given the multifactorial etiology of child obesity, it is unlikely that changing child care nutrition alone will be sufficient to improve young children's nutrition and weight status. However, the growing number of children in child care for long periods of the day warrants the adoption of optimal nutrition standards by licensed child care facilities.

ble 4. Child care nutrition standards for toddlers (≥1 year old)

at foods should be served	
jetables	Offer vegetables ≥2 times per day Vegetables can be fresh, frozen, or canned (all with no added salt, sugar, or fat) Offer dark green, orange, red, or deep yellow vegetables ≥1 time per day Do not serve deep-fried or prefried baked vegetables
its	Offer fruit ≥2 times per day Offer only fruit that is fresh, frozen, or canned in water (all with no added sugars)
teins	Do not serve processed meat or deep-fried or prefried meat or fish Offer lean protein ≥2 times per day, such as seafood, fish, lean meat, poultry, eggs, beans, peas, soy products, tofu, or unsalted nuts/seeds Offer yogurt ≤1 time per day, must have <23 g sugar per 6 oz Offer natural cheese ≤1–2 times per day; choose low-fat or reduced-fat cheese; do not serve cheese food/spread Serve protein foods with no added salt
ins	Offer whole grains most of the time Limit offering white (non-whole) grains Avoid offering white grain-based desserts
verages	Do not serve sugar-sweetened beverages Rarely or never offer 100% fruit juice When offered, give ≤1 age-appropriate serving of 100% fruit juice per day Ensure that water is easily available for self-serve indoors and outdoors and actively offered with meals and snacks and at other times as appropriate Offer unflavored whole milk ≥2 times per day for children 12–24 months Offer unflavored fat-free (also called nonfat or skim) or 1% (also called low-fat) milk ≥2 times per day for children >24 months Offer only nondairy milk substitutions (e.g., soy milk) that are nutritionally equivalent to milk[1]
jar, sodium, d fat	Do not serve foods with added sugar or sugar equivalents (e.g., high-fructose corn syrup, fructose, corn syrup, cane sugar, evaporated cane juice, or sucrose) listed as the first or second ingredients or having a combination of ≥3 kinds of sugar/sugar equivalents Do not serve low-calorie sweeteners or items containing low-calorie sweeteners (e.g., diet foods or diet beverages) Do not serve high-salt foods (>200 mg sodium per snack item or >480 mg sodium per entrée) Do not add salt at the table Use only liquid nontropical vegetable oils instead of solid fats
v foods should be served	
ing quency	Offer ≥1 meal and 1 snack for care <8 h Offer ≥2 meals and 2 snacks for care ≥8 h Provide meals and snacks every 2–3 h at regularly scheduled times
al and ack times	Serve family style meals and snacks; providers teach children to serve themselves age-appropriate portion sizes with assistance as needed Use dishware and utensils that are sized appropriately At least 1 child care provider sits with children at a table and eats the same meals and snacks Allow enough time to eat Provider models healthy eating and does not consume other items in front of the children Offer a variety of culturally relevant items Avoid choking hazards (e.g., by cutting grapes into smaller pieces and avoiding certain foods like nuts) When food is provided at celebrations or fundraisers offer only healthy items, such as fruit, vegetables, whole grains, low-fat dairy products, lean proteins, and water

Table 4 (continued)

Self-regulation	Do not use foods or beverages as reward or punishment or for comfort Ask children if they are full before removing plates and ask if they are hungry before serving seconds Expect young children to eat a lot of some meals and very little of others and to be messy; it may take months or years to accept new foods Expect children to not eat everything offered and to change likes/dislikes Do not pressure children to eat or clean their plates Mealtime conversations should not focus on the amount of food that is or is not eaten Minimize distractions while eating (e.g., no TV, toys, phones, or video games)

[1] Information on soy equivalents to milk can be accessed at: https://wicworks.fns.usda.gov/wicworks/Learning_Center/soybeverage.pdf.

The infant and toddler nutrition standards developed through review of authoritative standards and ranking by research and practice-experienced specialists have the potential to influence children in licensed family child care homes and centers in the USA. In addition, the process used to develop the standards may be adapted to establish or refine nutrition standards for child care settings in other countries. These standards should next be tested in a randomized controlled intervention trial in the USA to assess both the feasibility for providers and the impact on child nutrition and weight. A number of communities that are focused on improving early childhood nutrition may welcome the opportunity to implement the standards voluntarily. The recommended standards may also inspire quality indicator-focused child care leaders to incorporate the science- and practice-based nutrition standards into their own efforts. Further, the standards could be used to inform the establishment of state-based policy tied to child care licensing or through training and technical assistance for providers. Given the large and growing number of young children in child care, improving nutrition of infants and toddlers in child care settings has the potential to reduce child obesity and improve child health.

Conflict of Interest Statement

The authors declare that there are no conflicts of interest.

References

1 Fryar CD, Carroll MD, Ogden CL: Health E-Stats: Prevalence of Overweight, Obesity, and Severe Obesity among Children and Adolescents Aged 2–19 Years: United States, 1963–1965 through 2015–2016. Atlanta, National Center for Health Statistics, Centers for Disease Control and Prevention, 2018. https://www.cdc.gov/nchs/data/hestat/obesity_child_15_16/obesity_child_15_16.pdf.

2 Saavedra JM, Deming D, Dattilo A, Reidy K: Lessons from the Feeding Infants and Toddlers Study in North America: what children eat, and implications for obesity prevention. Ann Nutr Metab 2013;62:27–36.

3 May L, Borger C, Weinfield N, et al: WIC Infant and Toddler Feeding Practices Study-2: Infant Year Report. Prepared by Westat under contract No. AG-3198-K-11-0073. Alexandria, US Department of Agriculture, Food, and Nutrition Service (Project Officer: Allison Magness), 2017. https://www.fns.usda.gov/wic/wic-infant-and-toddler-feeding-practices-study-2-infant-year-report.

4 Au LE, Gurzo K, Paolicelli C, et al: Diet quality of US infants and toddlers 7–24 months old in the WIC Infant and Toddler Feeding Practices Study-2. J Nutr 2018;148:1786–1793.

5 Welker EB, Jacquier EF, Catellier DJ, et al: Room for improvement remains in food consumption patterns of young children aged 2–4 years. J Nutr 2018;148:1536S–1546S.

6 Borger C, Weinfield N, Zimmerman T, et al: WIC Infant and Toddler Feeding Practices Study-2: Second Year Report. Prepared by Westat under contract No. AG-3198-K-11-0073. Alexandria, US Department of Agriculture, Food, and Nutrition Service (Project Officer: Courtney Paolicelli), 2018. https://www.fns.usda.gov/wic/wic-infant-and-toddler-feeding-practices-study-2-second-year-report.

7 US Department of Health and Human Services and US Department of Agriculture: 2015–2020 Dietary Guidelines for Americans, Eighth Edition. Office of Disease Prevention and Health Promotion, 2015. https://health.gov/our-work/food-and-nutrition/2015-2020-dietary-guidelines/.

8 US Department of Labor: Facts Over Time – Women in the Labor Force. Washington, Women's Bureau, 2016. https://www.dol.gov/agencies/wb/data/facts-over-time/women-in-the-labor-force

9 US Bureau of Labor Statistics: Families with Own Children: Employment Status of Parents by Age of Youngest Child and Family Type, 2017–2018 Annual Averages. Washington, US Bureau of Labor Statistics, 2020. https://www.bls.gov/news.release/famee.t04.htm.

10 Laughlin L: Who's Minding the Kids? Child Care Arrangements. Current Population Reports. Washington, US Bureau of the Census. 2013. https://www.census.gov/prod/2013pubs/p70-135.pdf.

11 Dixon LB, Breck A, Khan LK: Comparison of children's food and beverage intakes with national recommendations in New York City child-care centers. Public Health Nutr 2016;19:2451–2457.

12 Alberdi G, McNamara AE, Lindsay KL, et al: The association between childcare and risk of childhood overweight and obesity in children aged 5 years and under: a systematic review. Eur J Pediatr 2016;175:1277–1294.

13 Black L, Matvienko-Sikar K, Kearney PM: The association between childcare arrangements and risk of overweight and obesity in childhood: a systematic review. Obes Rev 2017;18:1170–1190.

14 Costa S, Adams J, Gonzalez-Nahm S, Benjamin Neelon SE: Childcare in infancy and later obesity: a narrative review of longitudinal studies. Curr Pediatr Rep 2017;5:118–131.

15 Kim J, Peterson K: Association of infant child care with infant feeding practices and weight gain among US infants. Arch Pediatr Adolesc Med 2008;162:627–633.

16 US Department of Agriculture Food and Nutrition Service: Nutrition Standards for CACFP Meals and Snacks. Child and Adult Care Food Program: Meal Pattern Revisions Related to the Healthy, Hunger-Free Kids Act of 2010. Final Rule. Washington, US Department of Agriculture Food and Nutrition Service, 2015. https://www.federalregister.gov/documents/2015/01/15/2015-00446/child-and-adult-care-food-program-meal-pattern-revisions-related-to-the-healthy-hunger-free-kids-act.

17 Homel Vitale E: Access to Food in Early Care Continues to Decline. California Food Policy Advocates. 2019. https://cfpa.net/access-to-food-in-early-care-continues-to-decline/.

18 Public Health Law Center: Healthy Eating, Active Play, Screen Time Best Practices: Child Care Licensing Laws. Saint Paul, Public Health Law Center, 2017. https://www.publichealthlawcenter.org/heal/ChildCareMaps.html.

19 Gonzalez-Nahm S, Grossman ER, Frost N, Benjamin-Neelon SE: Early feeding in child care in the United States: are state regulations supporting breastfeeding? Prev Med 2017;105:232–236.

20 Benjamin-Neelon SE, Gonzalez-Nahm S, Grossman E, et al: State variations in infant feeding regulations for child care. Pediatrics 2017;140:e20172076.

21 Monsivais P, Johnson DB: Improving nutrition in home child care: are food costs a barrier? Public Health Nutr 2012;15:370–376.

22 US Department of Health and Human Services, Administration for Children and Families: Characteristics of Home-Based Early Care and Education Providers: Initial Findings from the National Survey of Early Care and Education. Washington, Office of Planning, Research and Evaluation, 2016. https://www.acf.hhs.gov/sites/default/files/opre/characteristics_of_home_based_early_care_and_education_toopre_032416.pdf.
23 Lee DL, Gurzo K, Yoshida S, et al: Compliance with the new 2017 Child and Adult Care Food Program standards for infants and children before implementation. Child Obes 2018;14:393–402.
24 Benjamin Neelon SE, Briley ME: Position of the American Dietetic Association: benchmarks for nutrition in child care. J Am Diet Assoc 2011;111:607–615.
25 Benjamin SE, Neelon B, Ball SC, et al: Reliability and validity of a nutrition and physical activity environmental self-assessment for child care. Int J Behav Nutr Phys Act 2007;4:29.
26 Institute of Medicine: Child and Adult Care Food Program: Aligning Dietary Guidance for All. Washington, The National Academies Press, 2011. https://www.nap.edu/catalog/12959/child-and-adult-care-food-program-aligning-dietary-guidance-for.
27 American Academy of Pediatrics, American Public Health Association, and National Resource Center for Health and Safety in Child Care and Early Education: Caring for Our Children: National Health and Safety Performance Standards; Guidelines for Early Care and Education Programs, ed 3. Elk Grove Village/Washington, American Academy of Pediatrics/American Public Health Association, 2011. https://nrckids.org/files/CFOC3_updated_final.pdf.
28 Nemours Foundation: Child Care Wellness Policy Workbook: Creating an Environment for Preschoolers to Develop Healthy Habits for Life. Nemours Foundation, 2012. https://www.nemours.org/content/dam/nemours/wwwv2/filebox/service/healthy-living/growuphealthy/Child%20Care%20Wellness%20Policy%20Workbook.pdf.
29 Zhou YE, Emerson JS, Levine RS, et al: Childhood obesity prevention interventions in childcare settings: systematic review of randomized and nonrandomized controlled trials. Am J Health Promot 2014;28:e92–e103.
30 van de Kolk I, Verjans-Janssen SRB, Gubbels JS, et al: Systematic review of interventions in the childcare setting with direct parental involvement: effectiveness on child weight status and energy balance-related behaviours. Int J Behav Nutr Phys Act 2019;16:110.

Published online: November 4, 2020

Black MM, Singhal A, Hillman CH (eds): Building Future Health and Well-Being of Thriving Toddlers and Young Children. Nestlé Nutr Inst Workshop Ser. Basel, Karger, 2020, vol 95, pp 67–77 (DOI: 10.1159/000511507)

Selected Micronutrient Needs of Children 1–3 Years of Age

Steven A. Abrams

Department of Pediatrics, Dell Medical School at the University of Texas, Austin, TX, USA

Abstract

Establishing dietary recommendations for micronutrients in young children is difficult. Techniques used to evaluate nutrient intake and bioavailability are hard to apply in this age group. Additionally, large variations in growth rates, dietary patterns, and nutrient losses in early childhood make determinations of dietary requirements difficult. Most recent studies have utilized stable isotopes to determine mineral absorption for iron, zinc, calcium, and magnesium. Vitamin D requirements have been established based on the dietary intake required to maintain a presumed adequate serum 25-hydroxyvitamin D concentration. Comparisons of nutrient requirements established using factorial methods involving absorption determinations and usual population intake are important to identify nutrients of concern related to deficient or excess intakes. Generally, in the USA, the intakes of calcium and magnesium are adequate to meet requirements in most toddler diets which include a milk source or a mineral-fortified milk alternative. Zinc and iron intakes can be below requirements in a substantial proportion of toddlers throughout the world, especially those with minimal meat consumption. Dietary vitamin D is generally below dietary recommendations, but clearly deficient serum 25-hydroxyvitamin D concentrations are less common, and the global role for routine vitamin D supplementation or fortification of the diet remains uncertain.

Introduction

Children 1–3 years of age (henceforth referred to by the imprecise, but commonly used term "toddlers") are among the most nutritionally understudied population. Techniques to assess micronutrients used in both younger and older age groups, including blood levels, mass balance studies, and isotopic techniques, are extremely difficult to apply to an age group that cannot directly consent to these procedures. It can be difficult to have families or regulatory oversight committees agree to what are perceived to be invasive research protocols with no direct benefit for the healthy children involved in them.

As such, data are very limited, and often only 1 or 2 studies in the last 30 years or more are available to directly evaluate this population. This is unfortunate as this is an age of important neurocognitive and motor development, and nutrient adequacy is critical. Most recent studies, especially of minerals, have used stable isotopes to assess nutrient absorption and metabolism. These techniques are safe although blood drawing and intravenous tracer infusions are not entirely noninvasive [1]. However, some important minerals in this age group, such as phosphorus, do not have minor stable isotopes that can be used as tracers, and others, including many vitamins, have poorly defined endpoints for nutritional adequacy or excess.

In this report, nutrient requirements of key micronutrients needed for growth and development of toddlers will be discussed. These are iron and zinc, critically needed for neurodevelopment, growth, and immune functioning, and calcium, vitamin D, and magnesium, related primarily to bone health. We will evaluate the current dietary recommendations for these nutrients, how these were determined, and how they relate to estimates of usual nutrient intake.

Methods to Assess Micronutrient Requirements

For the minerals, the technique most widely used in recent decades has been the factorial method in which nutrient needs for growth and recovery of losses are compared to intake-adjusted bioavailability using stable isotopes. For calcium, data for growth requirements are derived from relatively recent bone mineral content studies, but for most minerals growth needs were calculated based on very limited data from cadaver studies primarily performed in the first half of the 20th century.

For iron, the stable isotope methodology of determining absorption, derived from earlier radioactive isotope techniques, relies on the incorporation of an orally administered iron isotope (often given with an enhancer of iron absorption such as vitamin C or with a meal) in red blood cells at 14–28 days [2, 3]. Interpretation of these findings includes evaluation both of the iron source and the relationship between the iron intake and the iron status, frequently assessed using serum ferritin, of the child. This technique is well described and has the benefit of being relatively easily adapted to research settings throughout the world.

For zinc, calcium, and magnesium, the preferred mineral absorption technique is the dual tracer study in which one stable isotope is administered orally, and a different one is given intravenously with primary analysis of absorption based on the relative enrichment of recovered isotopes in the urine [4–6]. This technique is more challenging for use in toddlers due to the difficulty both in administering the isotope intravenously and in collecting multiple or extended urine specimens. Nonetheless, some studies have been performed although further data are critically needed, especially in nonindustrialized nations. A significant ongoing limitation to further expansion of this research is the cost of the isotopes themselves as well as the cost and limited availability of sites capable of accurate analysis of biological samples enriched in mineral-stable isotopes.

Assessing usual nutrient intake to determine the relationship between identified nutrient intake requirements and usual population intakes is also challenging in toddlers. The diet in this age group is often highly variable. It is not simple to have parents accurately recall or measure dietary intake, and no real nutritional steady state is generally feasible prior to conducting short-term isotopic absorption studies. Fortunately, with these limitations in mind, in addition to the National Health and Nutrition Examination Survey (NHANES), there are multiple datasets available recently in the USA and throughout the world that can be used to assess usual intake, although, as with absorption studies, more data are needed from nonindustrialized countries [7–12].

These data limitations are important in interpreting dietary recommendations [13–16]. It is not reasonable to be overprecise in interpreting recommendations and their relationship with usual intakes of populations of toddlers. Analysis of the proportion of the population below or above a threshold is often an inadequate way to determine nutrient adequacy in the face of severe limitations in the precision and accuracy of the data. Disease-oriented outcomes, including rickets for example, reflect extremely deficient outcomes in most cases and are often unreliable markers of population nutrient adequacy.

Fig. 1. Metabolism of dietary iron by toddlers. About 18% of overall iron is absorbed to meet tissue needs of an average of 0.6 mg/day.

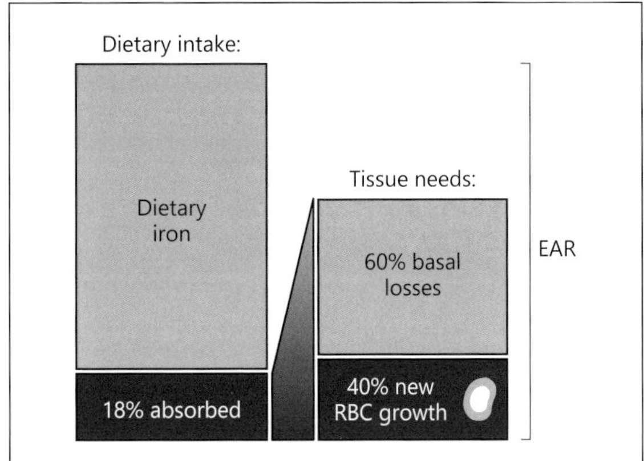

Specific Nutrients

Iron

The recommended intakes for iron have been set using a factorial approach in which the mean requirement of toddlers is about 0.6 mg/day of absorbed iron and the 97th percentile of this requirement is 1.2 mg/day. Of note is that about 60% of the requirement is related to basal iron losses – not growth needs for new red blood cell production (Fig. 1). The Institute of Medicine then used an approximate absorption fraction of 18% to calculate an estimated average requirement (EAR) for iron of 3 mg/day and a recommended dietary allowance (RDA) of 7 mg/day [13]. These values are relatively similar to those determined by the European Food Safety Authority (EFSA) of 5 and 7 mg/day, respectively, for the equivalent requirements [16].

In comparing these values to usual intakes on a global basis, it appears that the mean daily intake of iron in the USA, Mexico, Europe, and Australia is about 7–10 mg consistent with most children in these locations having intakes above the EAR [7–10, 12]. In contrast, lower daily intake with a mean of about 5 mg was reported in the Philippines [11]. In the USA, about one-fourth of toddlers have an intake below the RDA suggesting that there remains a subset of toddlers in whom further efforts to ensure adequate intake is indicated [8].

Of concern is that, globally, the prevalence of anemia remains very high with large differences between regions, ranging from about 20 to nearly 70%. Assuming that 30–50% of this anemia is related to iron deficiency, it may be that the factorial calculation used to determine dietary recommendations underestimates the biological need in this population [17, 18]. If this is the case, both higher basal iron loss rates and lower bioavailability from typical diets than the 18% used to calculate the dietary reference intake values are likely responsible.

Table 1. Summary of key current considerations: iron and zinc

Iron	In industrialized countries, intake matches published requirements for most small children; this is less true for nonindustrialized countries, and significant shortfalls and anemia persist in all locations The huge variation in iron bioavailability from dietary sources indicates that the use of one population standard for targeted intake may not be useful, and vigilance is needed to identify individuals or populations with low-bioavailable iron sources in their diet and at risk of iron deficiency despite seemingly adequate intake
Zinc	Generally, intakes are well above recommendations for most toddlers; as with iron, this is truer in industrialized settings Zinc needs to be considered in concert with iron and other minerals, including copper, in determining fortification and supplementation strategies Dietary concerns about exceeding upper dietary reference intake levels are likely not a reason to lower current fortification strategies, but further data are needed

When we evaluated iron bioavailability in a population of small children in Mexico, we found huge variability in absorption efficiency depending on the iron compound and whether it was provided with vitamin C [3]. This range in absorption (from 1 to 24% of intake) highlights the need to focus not just on usual population daily intakes for iron but also on the iron source and other dietary components.

Zinc

Consideration of zinc requirements has focused both on the RDA but also on the limits of intake, referred to as the tolerable upper limit (UL). The EAR for zinc has been set as 2.5 mg/day in the USA/Canada and the equivalent value of 3.6 mg/day in Europe [13, 15]. The RDA for zinc has been set for this age group at 3 mg/day in the USA/Canada and 4.3 mg/day for Europe [13, 15]. Our studies in this population using stable isotopes tend to support the EFSA value for average requirement although it is difficult to be precise as relatively few toddlers have these very low iron intakes in the USA [5]. Regardless of the exact EAR recommended, the EAR is well below the usual intakes in the USA, Canada, and Mexico of about 6–8 mg/day [7, 8].

This usual intake level has prompted concerns as the USA and Canada UL is 7 mg/day, implying that a large proportion of toddlers may have high zinc intakes leading to a risk of toxicity, potentially related to a diminished copper status [13]. Numerous groups have challenged this UL as not reflective of dietary sources of zinc and copper, and recently the izincg collaborate has suggested that a no adverse effect level of 10 mg/day in toddlers 1–3 years old is more appropriate [19], and the World Health Organization (WHO) sets a UL value of 23 mg/day [20]. There is little if any evidence that usual diets including high-zinc-containing natural dietary sources, such as red meat, lead to deficiencies in other

Table 2. Approximate calcium content of typical beverages for toddlers

Beverage	Calcium concentration	Daily intake, per 500 mL/day
Breast milk	26 mg/100 mL	130 mg
Whole cow's milk	120 mg/100 mL	600 mg
Fortified rice/soy/almond milk[1]	20 mg/100 mL	600 mg
Toddler "formula"[2]	110 mg/100 mL	550 mg
Goat milk	130 mg/100 mL	650 mg
Unfortified almond milk[1]	<10 mg	<10 mg
Unfortified soy milk[1]	25 mg	125 mg

[1] Many, but not all, soy- and other plant-based beverages commercially sold are calcium fortified.
[2] The World Health Organization and American Academy of Pediatrics do not recommend the use of these formulas.

micronutrients, although concern may exist when the zinc is taken as a supplement (Table 1) [21].

Calcium

Calcium dietary requirements have largely been set in childhood based on the usual rate at which the skeleton accretes calcium. Various estimates based largely on bone mineral mass accumulation data suggest this rate in toddlers is about 100 mg/day on average with a high end (97th percentile value) of about 140 mg/day. The EAR in the USA and Canada is 500 mg/day, and the RDA is 700 mg/day in this age group [22]. These values are consistent with a stable isotope study we conducted in toddlers evaluating calcium absorption and retention on a range of calcium intakes from about 100–1,000 mg/day [4].

Usual calcium intakes in the USA and Canada are above both the EAR and the RDA at about 950 mg/day although up to 20% of toddlers will be below the RDA [7, 8, 14]. This provides support for provision of high-calcium-containing dietary sources in this age group, with yogurts or similar foods containing naturally high calcium being considered for those toddlers whose primary non-water beverage source is breast milk or a non-calcium-fortified plant beverage (Table 2).

Vitamin D

It is impossible to consider dietary calcium requirements without consideration of vitamin D requirements, and these were considered together in the dietary reference intake process published by the Institute of Medicine in 2011 [14]. Although a full review of vitamin D needs of toddlers is beyond the scope of this review, a few key points are relevant. First, the outcome usually used to evaluate vitamin D status, the serum 25-hydroxyvitamin D (25-OHD) concentration, is not a full measure of the most clinically relevant outcome in toddlers preventing nutritional rickets. The complex relationship between calcium and vitamin D deficiency leading to rickets has been discussed in detail in several reviews [23, 24]. Although targeted levels of 25-OHD are usually set at 50 nmol/L, it is likely that calcium absorption is only substantially limited at lower levels, such as below 30 nmol/L [24, 25]. Whether other potential benefits, such as immune function, require higher 25-OHD levels remains uncertain, especially in small children.

A globally based approach to decreasing vitamin D deficiency has recently been published. Key issues are the use of national strategies related to food fortification and/or supplementation strategies with vitamin D. These may be best considered in countries in which 20% of the population at risk has a 25-OHD level below 30 nmol/L and/or a >1% prevalence of rickets [24]. This is consistent with a Cochrane review suggesting that supplementation of deficient children (approximately <35 nmol/L) may be useful, but that there are few data supporting supplementation strategies to improve bone density in healthy children with higher 25-OHD levels [26]. In the USA, <20% of the population has a 25-OHD level <50 nmol/L, and in Mexico a recent study found 25% <50 nmol/L [27]. Nonetheless, the persistence of clinical rickets in many parts of the world is consistent with careful vigilance, and there is little likelihood of harm in vitamin D fortification strategies for milk and other beverages.

Magnesium

The importance of magnesium for health outcomes is increasingly recognized in all age groups. However, although stable isotopic absorption studies are feasible for magnesium, they are technically more difficult than for calcium and zinc, and they have been very rarely performed in children. Furthermore, because toddlers only retain a very small amount of magnesium daily (about 10–20 mg), it is difficult to be precise about the relationship between dietary magnesium intake and net retention.

With these limitations in mind, we found that a dietary intake of about 100 mg/daily led to a net magnesium retention of about 20 mg/daily in toddlers. However, it is likely that 20 mg/day slightly exceeds the average typical magnesium retention in this age group. The EAR for magnesium was set at 65 mg and the RDA at 80 mg/day [28]. Although these values may be a bit low, it is important to note that the 1st percentile of usual magnesium intakes in the USA and Canada is 80 mg/day, and the median intake is 180 mg/day. These data suggest limited population-based concern in the USA related to magnesium dietary suf-

Table 3. Summary of key current considerations: bone minerals and vitamin D

Calcium	Likely average physiological need about 300–400 mg/day Easily achieved with diet that includes dairy or fortified plant or other beverages Breastfed toddlers should have adequate solid food or other dietary source of calcium Need to have awareness of this issue especially in vegan or other restrictive diets
Vitamin D	Related to bone health, there is a low but definite persistence of severe vitamin D deficiency in this age group, since dietary intakes are low in many populations Specific risk groups exist, and rickets remains a clinical problem especially when combined with low calcium intakes Global strategies and assessments are needed to evaluate the need for fortification and supplementation
Magnesium	No good biomarker exists for magnesium Limited accretion data suggest target retention of 10–20 mg/day in childhood Magnesium-deficient intake is likely relatively uncommon with mixed diets, but difficult for clinicians to assess No current recommendations for routine fortification or supplementation, but limited data available

ficiency, but further information would be needed on a global basis or related to the bioavailability of different magnesium sources. Of note is that in slightly older, i.e., 4- to 8-year-old children, we found a closer relationship between dietary magnesium intake than dietary calcium intake for total body bone mineral content and density, further providing evidence that a closer look at the role of magnesium in bone health in small children should be undertaken (Table 3) [29].

Dietary Sources of Key Minerals and Fortification Strategies

The diet of toddlers is unique in that it represents a transition between that of infants, which is largely based on breast milk or formula with gradual introduction of solid foods, and that of older children, which at the end of the toddler age period begins to resemble the family diet.

With regard to minerals, in many countries, a key source of bone minerals and vitamins, including calcium, magnesium, and vitamin D, is cow's milk, or for families who do not use cow's milk, soy or other plant milks. Cow's milk is rich in these components and represents the major mineral source for them. Soy and other non-cow milks are often fortified with minerals to meet these needs. For toddlers who do not receive significant cow's milk or fortified plant milks, including those infants who are breastfed during the toddler age period, bone minerals, and especially vitamin D, may be minimal, and there may be some risk of rickets. In these cases, it is generally recommended to provide vitamin D via supplement. Calcium is less commonly given via supplement but is found in foods, such as corn tortillas prepared from lime treatment. We evaluated calcium absorption from these tortillas with stable isotopes and found a high rate of absorption [30]. Generally, calcium is less likely to be fortified in foods such as flour than other minerals, but this can be done in high-risk populations, or supplements can be provided where the rate of rickets related to mineral deficiency is substantial. Attention needs to be paid related to other components of the diet including levels of phytates, which may affect calcium absorption as well as that of other minerals [31].

Dietary iron sources including fortified foods are a critical issue especially in populations with high rates of iron deficiency. A detailed review of this topic is beyond the scope of this review, but a critical issue as noted above is the form of the iron provided and its bioavailability. The diet of toddlers is often very low in meat, and fortification of grains is therefore widely done both for iron and zinc. Critical issues also include the iron:zinc ratio in the fortificants and the specific method of preparation of the fortified food. Of importance is that when fortification strategies do not include a careful evaluation of iron bioavailability, they may not achieve desired results [3, 32]. Nonetheless, fortification strategies remain a central pillar of nutritional programming in many countries related to the iron needs of toddlers.

Future Research Needs

Determination of dietary requirements for vitamins and minerals in small children requires accurate evaluation of usual intakes, mineral absorption efficiency, and excretion along with an assessment of an outcome measure that is biologically meaningful. The lack of adequate data in this age group for each of these should be addressed with specific research targeting this population. This effort needs to be global in scope and to fully account for differences in dietary patterns that are regional or cultural in nature. Overemphasis on very specific values for dietary recommendations may lead to unnecessary interventions, and the risks and benefits of nutrient supplementation and fortification strategies need to be assessed broadly.

Acknowledgment

The author would like to acknowledge Hannah R. Abrams, MD, for preparing the figure used in the manuscript.

Conflict of Interest Statement

Dr. Abrams received no funding and accepted no honorarium for this paper.

References

1 Abrams SA: Using stable isotopes to assess mineral absorption and utilization by children. Am J Clin Nutr 1999;70:955–964.

2 Lynch MF, Griffin IJ, Hawthorne KM, et al: Iron absorption is more closely related to iron status than daily iron intake in 12- to 48-mo-old children. J Nutr 2007:137:88–92.

3 Pérez-Expósito AB, Villalpando S, Rivera JA, et al: Ferrous sulfate is more bioavailable among preschoolers than other forms of iron in a milk-based weaning food distributed by PROGRESA – a national program in Mexico. J Nutr 2005;135:64–69.

4 Lynch MF, Griffin IJ, Hawthorne KM, et al: Calcium balance in 1–4-y-old children. Am J Clin Nutr 2007;85:750–754.

5 Griffin IJ, Lynch MF, Hawthorne KM, et al: Zinc homeostasis in 1–4 year olds consuming diets typical of US children. Br J Nutr 2007;98:358–363.

6 Griffin IJ, Lynch MF, Hawthorne KM, et al: Magnesium retention in 12–48 mo-old children. J Am Coll Nutr 2008;27:349–355.

7 Eldridge AL, Catellier DJ, Hampton JC, et al: Trends in mean nutrient intakes of US infants, toddlers, and young children from 3 Feeding Infants and Toddlers Studies (FITS). J Nutr 2019; 149:1230–1237.

8 Hamner HC, Perrine CG, Scanlon KS: Usual intake of key minerals among children in the second year of life, NHANES 2003–2012. Nutrients 2016;8:468.

9 Sánchez-Pimienta TG, López-Olmedo N, Rodríguez-Ramírez S, et al: High prevalence of inadequate calcium and iron intakes by Mexican population groups as assessed by 24-hour recalls. J Nutr 2016;146:1874S–1880S.

10 Scott JA, Gee G, Devenish G, et al: Determinants and sources of iron intakes of Australian toddlers: findings from the SMILE cohort study. Int J Environ Res Public Health 2019;16:E181.

11 Denney L, Angeles-Agdeppa I, Capanzana MV, et al: Nutrient intakes and food sources of Filipino infants, toddlers and young children are inadequate: findings from the National Nutrition Survey 2013. Nutrients 2018;10:E1730.

12 van der Merwe LF, Eussen SR: Iron status of young children in Europe. Am J Clin Nutr 2017; 106:1663S–1671S.

13 Institute of Medicine, Food and Nutrition Board: Dietary Reference Intakes for Vitamin A, Vitamin K, Arsenic, Boron, Chromium, Copper, Iodine, Iron, Manganese, Molybdenum, Nickel, Silicon, Vanadium, and Zinc. Washington, National Academies Press, 2001.

14 IOM (Institute of Medicine). Dietary Reference Intakes for Vitamin D and Calcium. Washington, National Academies Press, 2011.

15 EFSA (European Food Safety Authority): Scientific opinion on dietary reference values for zinc. EFSA J 2014;12:3844 (revised 2015).

16 EFSA (European Food Safety Authority): Dietary reference values for nutrients: summary report. EFSA Supp Publ 2017;14:e15121. https://doi.org/10.2903/sp.efsa.2017.e15121.

17 Miller JL: Iron deficiency anemia: a common and curable disease. Cold Spring Harb Perspect Med 2013;3:a011866.

18 McLean E, Cogswell M, Egli I, et al: Worldwide prevalence of anaemia, WHO Vitamin and Mineral Nutrition Information System, 1993–2005. Public Health Nutr 2009;12:444–454.

19 IZiNCG Symposium Presentations. 2010. https://www.izincg.org/symposium-presentations.

20 Gibson RS, King JC, Lowe N: A review of dietary zinc recommendations. Food Nutr Bull 2016;37: 443–460.

21 Olivares M, Pizarro F, López de Romaña D: Effect of zinc sulfate fortificant on iron absorption from low extraction wheat flour co-fortified with ferrous sulfate. Biol Trace Elem Res 2013;151:471–475.

22 Peacock M: Calcium absorption efficiency and calcium requirements in children and adolescents. Am J Clin Nutr 1991;54:261S–265S.

23 Carpenter TO, Shaw NJ, Portale AA, et al: Rickets. Nat Rev Dis Primers 2017;3:17101.

24 Roth DE, Abrams SA, Aloia J, et al: Global prevalence and disease burden of vitamin D deficiency: a roadmap for action in low- and middle-income countries. Ann N Y Acad Sci 2018;1430:44–79.

25 Abrams SA, Hicks PD, Hawthorne KD: Higher serum 25-hydroxyvitamin D levels in school-age children are inconsistently associated with increased calcium absorption. J Clin Endocrinol Metab 2009;94:2421–2427.

26 Winzenberg T, Powell S, Shaw KA, Jones G: Effects of vitamin D supplementation on bone density in healthy children: systematic review and meta-analysis. BMJ 2011;342:c7254.

27 Flores M, Macias N, Lozada A, et: Serum 25-hydroxyvitamin D levels among Mexican children ages 2 y to 12 y: a national survey. Nutrition 2013;29:802–804.
28 Institute of Medicine, Food and Nutrition Board: Dietary Reference Intakes for Calcium, Magnesium, Phosphorus, Vitamin D, and Fluoride. Washington, National Academies Press, 1997.
29 Abrams SA, Chen Z, Hawthorne KM: Magnesium metabolism in 4-year-old to 8-year-old children. J Bone Miner Res 2014;29:118–122.
30 Rosado JL, Diaz M, Rosas A, et al: Calcium absorption from corn tortilla is relatively high and is dependent upon calcium content and liming in Mexican women. J Nutr 2005;135:2578–2581.
31 Thacher TD, Aliu O, Griffin IJ, et al: Meals and dephytinization affect calcium and zinc absorption in Nigerian children with rickets. J Nutr 2009;139:926–932.
32 Walter T, Pizarro F, Abrams SA, Boy E: Bioavailability of elemental iron powder in white wheat bread. Eur J Clin Nutr 2004;58:555–558.

Published online: November 9, 2020

Black MM, Singhal A, Hillman CH (eds): Building Future Health and Well-Being of Thriving Toddlers and Young Children. Nestlé Nutr Inst Workshop Ser. Basel, Karger, 2020, vol 95, pp 78–87 (DOI: 10.1159/000511516)

You Are What Your Parents Eat: Parental Influences on Early Flavor Preference Development

Catherine A. Forestell

Department of Psychological Sciences, The College of William & Mary, Williamsburg, VA, USA

Abstract

To understand the development of children's flavor preferences, it is important to consider the context of the feeding environment. Although children are predisposed to prefer sweet-tasting foods and beverages and to avoid bitter-tasting foods such as dark-green vegetables, parents can play a central role in shifting these innate food acceptance patterns throughout development. Beginning before birth, the fetus detects the continually changing flavor profile of amniotic fluid, which reflects the mother's diet. After birth, if mothers choose to breastfeed, these sensory experiences continue. Through this process of familiarization, women who maintain a healthy diet throughout pregnancy and lactation prepare their infants to like healthful foods. Upon the introduction of solid foods, repeated exposure to a variety of healthful foods promotes acceptance for these foods and for novel foods. In addition to providing sensory exposures to a range of healthful foods, parents can shape children's flavor preferences by modeling healthy eating behaviors and by creating supportive feeding environments. The degree to which parents engage in these practices is influenced by demographic and societal characteristics. Considering the context in which children and families live will encourage the development of evidence-based strategies that more effectively support children's healthy eating habits.

Introduction

Children consume fewer fruits and vegetables than recommended, and their diets are high in saturated fat, sugar, and salt. In the USA, more than 25% of toddlers do not consume a single serving of fruits or vegetables on any given day [1], and their consumption of sweet and salty snacks and sugar-sweetened beverages is rising [2]. The preference for simple sugars and energy-dense foods over nutrient-rich alternatives has a variety of serious health consequences, such as type 2 diabetes, cardiovascular disease, and heightened risk of obesity. Because the first 1,000 days of life are considered a critical period for obesity prevention efforts [3], it is important to understand the factors that are related to the development of early preferences for nutritious, healthful foods.

Children's unhealthy dietary preferences reflect their basic biology. As previously reviewed [4], heightened preference for intense sweetness and rejection of bitter tastes are innate and considered to be a hallmark of youth. Within hours of birth, infants demonstrate a preference for sweet taste. They consume more of a sweet-tasting liquid relative to plain water [5], and they display facial expressions of relaxation and pleasure in response to a sweetened solution placed on the tongue [6]. Although preference for sweet taste remains elevated throughout childhood, it begins to decline in adolescence [7]. In contrast, children's response to bitter-tasting foods is decidedly negative. For example, neonates respond with gapes, nose wrinkles, and frowns after a small amount of a bitter solution is placed in the oral cavity [6]. Beginning around 2 weeks of age, infants consume less of a bitter-tasting urea solution relative to water [8]. Infant's rejection of bitter tastes, which continues throughout childhood, explains why they often refuse to eat many vegetables, particularly those of the *Brassica* genus (e.g., broccoli or Brussels sprouts), which are high in bitter polyphenols.

These responses seem maladaptive in today's society where we have easy access to tasty, energy-dense foods. However, if we consider taste perception from an evolutionary perspective, its adaptive role becomes apparent. Acceptance of sweet taste likely evolved to enhance survival in an environment where nutrients and sources of energy were scarce, thereby attracting children to available sources of nutrients and energy during periods of maximal growth. In contrast, perception and dislike of bitter taste may have evolved to protect against the high risk of accidentally ingesting lethal toxins which often taste bitter [9]. Although early preference for sweet taste and avoidance of bitter taste is inborn, an important feature of the gustatory system is that it is inherently plastic, especially during infancy and childhood. Consequently, children can learn to like bitter foods through early sensory experiences.

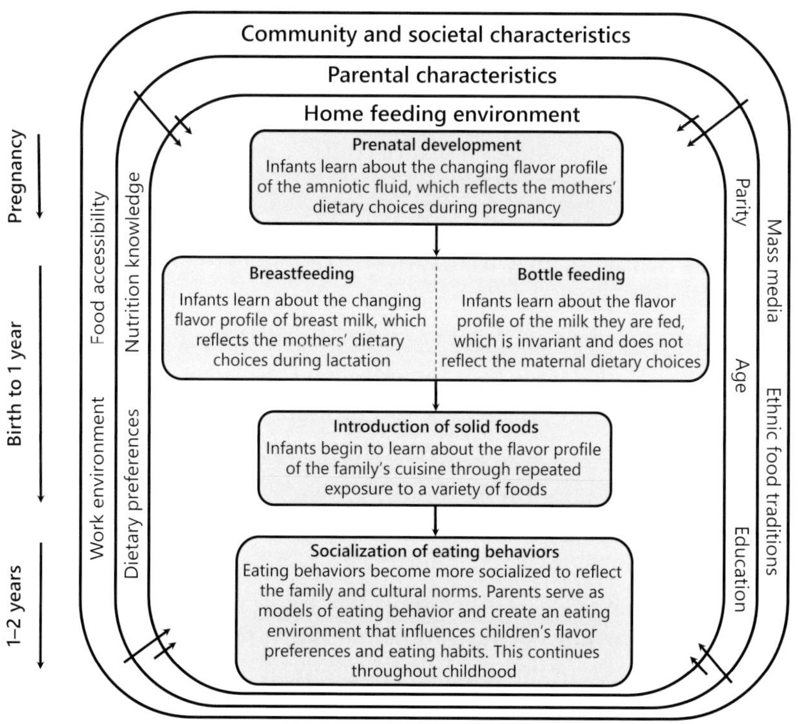

Fig. 1. Depiction of the young child's feeding environment within the context of the family, which is influenced by various community and societal characteristics.

Parents' dietary habits shape the availability of and accessibility to foods in the home [10], and, as a result, they play a central role in providing early sensory experiences that cultivate children's palates. With this in mind, the goal of this paper is to review recent research with a focus on the role of parents in the development of children's early flavor preferences, especially for bitter green vegetables. I will focus on flavor learning over the first 1,000 days, beginning with conception until the end of the second year of life. As will be reviewed below, evidence suggests that a range of external factors, such as culture, socioeconomic status, and food availability, influences dietary choices that parents make for themselves and for their families (Fig. 1). As a result, these factors should be considered when developing evidence-based strategies that endeavor to increase bitter green vegetable acceptance and consumption in young children.

Perinatal Sensory Experiences and the Role of the Mother

Flavor experiences begin before birth with the emergence of the olfactory and gustatory systems. As reviewed in more detail elsewhere [11], by the last trimester, the taste and olfactory systems are functional and capable of detecting and communicating information to structures in the brain responsible for organizing and controlling affective behaviors. By term, infants are actively swallowing between 500 and 1,000 mL of amniotic fluid per day, which stimulates the taste buds and olfactory cells. The early development of the taste and olfactory systems allows infants to detect the continually changing flavor profile of the amniotic fluid. In addition to containing chemicals with distinct taste properties, a wide variety of volatile chemicals that are either ingested (e.g., fruits, vegetables, and spices) or inhaled (e.g., cigarette smoke) by the mother are transmitted to the amniotic fluid.

Research suggests that early sensory experiences that occur during pregnancy are encoded, and these memories subsequently play a role in the acceptance of solid foods (for a review see Spahn et al. [12]). Consistent evidence shows that prenatal flavor exposure increases acceptance of similarly flavored foods during infancy and childhood. Although more research is needed to investigate how long these early flavor memories facilitate food acceptance, one study has shown that prenatal flavor exposures may have long-term effects. In this study, 8- to 9-year-old children who were exposed prenatally to garlic ate a higher proportion of garlic-flavored compared to plain potato in a laboratory session compared to children who were not exposed to garlic prenatally [13].

After birth, infants' flavor experiences continue as they begin to consume either formula or breast milk. Compared to formula feeding, breastfeeding provides children with an advantage in developing preferences for healthy foods, especially if mothers have healthy dietary habits. Like that of amniotic fluid, the flavor profile of breast milk reflects the foods eaten by the mother and her culinary traditions. Exposure to flavors transmitted to breast milk from the mothers' diet facilitates infants' acceptance of solid foods. In a recent study, Mennella et al. [14] demonstrated that breastfed infants whose mothers consumed a variety of vegetable juices for 1 month during lactation were more accepting of carrot-flavored cereal relative to a control group of breastfed infants whose mothers avoided the vegetable juices. Earlier exposure to vegetables through mother's breast milk, beginning 2 weeks postpartum, was more effective than later exposure that began either 6 or 10 weeks postpartum. Other research has suggested that mothers' vegetable consumption during breastfeeding may have long-term consequences on flavor preference development. This was supported by a recent study of 1,396 mother-child dyads that controlled for socioeconomic status and fruit and vegetable availability during childhood [15]. This study reported that among children breastfed for at least 4 months, each additional serving of vegetables consumed by lactating mothers significantly increased the odds that vegetable consumption would be high (i.e., ≥1 daily serving) at 6 years of age. In combination, these studies suggest that mothers' vegetable consumption as well as a longer duration of breastfeeding may facilitate children's preferences throughout childhood.

Environmental Factors That Limit Newborns' Exposure to Flavors of Healthful Foods

The transition from pregnancy to the postpartum period may be associated with a negative impact on maternal dietary habits, especially in low-income women. Although women who breastfeed report higher fruit and vegetable intake than women who bottle feed [16], the prevalence of exclusive breastfeeding over the first 6 months of life is low in the USA. While more than two-thirds of women (81%) initiate breastfeeding at birth, only 20% are still breastfeeding by the time their child reaches 6 months of age. These statistics vary by racial background, with African American women experiencing some of the lowest breastfeeding rates nationally (i.e., 64% initiate breastfeeding and only 14% are exclusively breastfeeding at 6 months) [17]. One important reason for the cessation of breastfeeding before 6 months of age in the USA is that women often return to work only 2–3 months after the birth of the child. In an attempt to overcome this challenge, changes in federal policy over the past decade now require workplaces to provide lactation rooms for breastfeeding mothers. While this policy change has increased breastfeeding duration for some women, those who are more disadvantaged continue to experience workplace disparities that limit their ability to sustain breastfeeding [18].

In combination, these findings suggest that many infants in the USA do not experience the benefits associated with breastfeeding throughout the first 6 months of life. Evidence shows that education interventions as well as social support, regardless of whether it is from a family member, friend, health care provider, or the workplace, increase breastfeeding. However, more research is needed to identify effective system level policies and practices to increase rates of breastfeeding [19].

Parents' Role in Complementary Feeding

Although there is wide variation in the introduction of solid foods, parents are advised to introduce solid foods at around 6 months of age. During this new stage of feeding, interactions between the infant and the parent become increasingly interdependent and bidirectional. Healthy feeding practices during this period have positive short- and long-term effects on body composition and growth, neurodevelopment, and the development of healthy preferences for healthy foods [20].

During complementary feeding, parents continue to play a powerful role in shaping children's flavor preferences by determining which foods are available, and how they will be prepared and flavored. Through these early experiences, children learn about the sensory properties of foods and develop schemas about how an acceptable food should look, taste, and smell. As will be reviewed, laboratory-based studies have identified several strategies for promoting infants' and toddlers' preferences for vegetables.

Parents' Role in Providing Sensory Exposures during Complementary Feeding

During complementary feeding, continued and repeated exposure to the flavors of healthful foods promotes familiarization with their sensory properties and, in turn, enhances acceptance of these foods. It is important to note that the process of familiarizing children with healthful foods may require patience. Although children will easily accept energy-dense foods and beverages that are high in sugar and salt upon initial presentation, less palatable foods typically require more presentations before they are readily accepted. In a recent study, after 5 exposures to an artichoke purée, toddlers consumed more of this vegetable and continued to accept it when tested 5 weeks after the intervention [21]. This study also assessed the role of associative learning by comparing the effectiveness of repeated exposure to plain artichoke purée to that of a purée with calories (flavor-nutrient learning) or a sweet taste (flavor-flavor learning). Results indicated that flavor-nutrient and flavor-flavor pairings increased children's acceptance of the artichoke purée to the same extent as repeated exposure to the plain version [21]. Overall, studies that have compared effects of associative conditioning with repeated exposure during infancy have yielded mixed findings, with several studies suggesting that repeated exposure is just as effective as associative conditioning at increasing children's consumption of vegetables.

There is significant variation between cultures with respect to the timing of introducing vegetables. Recent research suggests that the order in which parents introduce fruits and vegetables may be important for long-term vegetable acceptance. In one example, infants were exclusively fed either vegetables or fruits during the first 2 weeks of complementary feeding. Several months later, when the infants were 12 months old, vegetable intake was 38% higher in those who were initially exposed to vegetables relative to those initially exposed to fruits [22]. These results, in combination with those from other studies, suggest that exposing children to vegetables early during complementary feeding may be an effective approach to increase later vegetable acceptance.

There is growing evidence that exposing infants and toddlers to a variety of vegetables is another effective method for increasing vegetable acceptance. A recent study showed that this approach may be especially effective for children who are weaned at around 6 months of age [23]. Infants who were either weaned between 4 and 5 months and those who were weaned between 5.5 and 6 months were exposed to 1 vegetable (carrots) or to a variety of vegetables (i.e., courgette, parsnip, or sweet potato) over 9 days. When infants were fed a novel vegetable (peas) in the test phase, those weaned after 5 months consumed significantly more after exposure to a variety of vegetables than those who were exposed to only 1 type of vegetable. In contrast, infants who were weaned earlier showed similar acceptance of the peas regardless of whether they had been fed a variety of vegetables or a single vegetable.

In combination, studies focused on complementary feeding suggest that to increase children's vegetable acceptance, mothers should introduce their infants to a wide range of vegetables and continue to offer those that are not initially accepted. Timing is also important, with evidence supporting early rather than later exposure to vegetables. Despite this scientific evidence, there is a wide range of attitudes and beliefs about solid food introduction across the world. For example, although vegetables are commonly the first food offered in many European countries, the types of vegetables offered are typically root vegetables, such as potatoes and carrots, rather than bitter green vegetables. In North America and Australia, more than half of children are initially fed infant cereals rather than vegetables [24]. Moreover, in North America, the commercial foods that are available for infants and toddlers may not promote the development of preferences for bitter green vegetables. A recent analysis of infant and toddler foods available in US supermarkets indicated that most single ingredient vegetables were red and orange vegetables. A minority of foods contained bitter green vegetables, such as spinach. In these foods, small quantities of green vegetables were mixed with more palatable vegetables or fruit [25].

Parents' Role in Socially Facilitating Flavor Preferences during Complementary Feeding

Although infants are relatively accepting of new foods soon after weaning, during the second year of life, they begin to become hesitant to accept new foods. This phenomenon, known as food neophobia, is associated with reduced fruit and vegetable acceptance and causes great frustration in parents. The feeding environment that parents create at this time sets the stage for the development of healthy flavor and food preferences that may eventually overcome neophobic responses [for a review, see ref. 26].

Parents can encourage children's healthy eating habits by employing an authoritative feeding style in which they take responsibility for their child's nutritional choices while providing a positive feeding environment that is supportive and responsive to the child's needs. In contrast, authoritarian feeding styles that involve coercive feeding practices are associated with more food refusals [27]. Infants and toddlers may also learn to associate foods with emotional tone of social interactions during feeding. For example, research with 3- to 4-year-old children has shown that repeated opportunities to taste a vegetable in a positive context where a parent praises the child for trying it increased its acceptance relative to repeated exposure alone [28]. Parental dietary habits also play an important role in encouraging acceptance of healthy foods. Ideally, if parents have a healthy diet themselves they will not only feed some of these foods to their toddlers, they will also model their own healthy eating habits. Children will try new foods more quickly and like healthful foods better when a parent models the consumption of those foods [29].

Environmental Limitations That Reduce Infants' and Toddlers' Access to Healthful Foods

One important factor that affects children's exposure to healthful foods in the home is the socioeconomic status of the family. Underprivileged families often have difficulty accessing and feeding healthy foods to their children because they live in areas that have limited access to nutritious foods, or they cannot afford to buy these foods. This issue combined with the short shelf life of fresh products or a lack of resources (such as a stove) to prepare the foods make it difficult to prepare meals that contain vegetables. To help mitigate some of these problems, the Special Supplemental Nutrition Program for Women, Infants, and Children (WIC) in the USA provides healthful foods and support services to low-income pregnant and postpartum women and their children up to 5 years of age. Although this program does not address all of the challenges listed above, WIC participation has been shown to increase children's consumption of green vegetables and lentils and decrease consumption of saturated fats over the first 2 years of life [30]. Moving forward, it will be important to develop and assess the effectiveness of additional interventions that involve tailored guidance and education about healthy eating to families.

Final Thoughts

From an early age, children learn how and what to eat, and develop expectations about how foods should look, taste, and smell. This learning occurs as a result of the interplay between children's biological predispositions, the food environment provided by their parents, and the community and culture in which they live. Mothers who consume an array of healthful foods throughout pregnancy and lactation – and who subsequently feed their children these foods during the complementary feeding period – can promote healthful eating habits in their children. However, due to a variety of social, economic, and cultural factors, parents vary dramatically in the food environment that they provide. Developing effective strategies that empower parents from all backgrounds to provide children with exposure to healthful foods in a supportive feeding environment is critical for promoting healthy dietary habits.

Conflict of Interest Statement

The author has no conflicts of interest to disclose related to the preparation of this article.

References

1 Miles G, Siega-Riz AM: Trends in food and beverage consumption among infants and toddlers: 2005–2012. Pediatrics 2017;139:e201632.
2 Piernas C, Popkin BM: Trends in snacking among US children. Health Aff (Millwood) 2010; 29:398–404.
3 Woo Baidal JA, Locks LM, Cheng ER, et al: Risk factors for childhood obesity in the first 1,000 days: a systematic review. Am J Prev Med 2016; 50:761–779.
4 Forestell CA: Flavor perception and preference development in human infants. Ann Nutr Metab 2017;70(S3):17–25.
5 Maller O, Turner RE: Taste in acceptance of sugars by human infants. J Comp Physiol Psychol 1973;84:496–501.
6 Steiner JE, Glaser D, Hawilo ME, Berridge KC: Comparative expression of hedonic impact: affective reactions to taste by human infants and other primates. Neurosci Biobehav Rev 2001;25:53–74.
7 Mennella JA, Lukasewycz LD, Griffith JW, Beauchamp GK: Evaluation of the Monell forced-choice, paired-comparison tracking procedure for determining sweet taste preferences across the lifespan. Chem Senses 2011;1;36:345–355.
8 Kajiura H, Cowart BJ, Beauchamp GK: Early developmental change in bitter taste responses in human infants. Dev Psychobiol 1992;25:375–386.
9 Glendinning JI: Is the bitter rejection response always adaptive? Physiol Behav 1994;56:1217–1227.
10 Robinson S, Marriott L, Poole J, et al; Southampton Women's Survey Study Group; Dietary patterns in infancy: the importance of maternal and family influences on feeding practice. Br J Nutr 2007;98:1029–1037.
11 Forestell CA, Mennella JA: The ontogeny of taste perception and preference throughout childhood; in Doty RL (ed): Handbook of Olfaction and Gustation, ed 3. New York, Dekker, 2015, pp 795–828.
12 Spahn JM, Callahan EH, Spill MK, et al: Influence of maternal diet on flavor transfer to amniotic fluid and breast milk and children's responses: a systematic review. Am J Clin Nutr 2019;109(S1): 1003S–1026S.
13 Hepper PG, Wells DL, Dornan JC, Lynch C: Long-term flavor recognition in humans with prenatal garlic experience. Dev Psychobiol 2013;55:568–574.
14 Mennella JA, Daniels LM, Reiter AR: Learning to like vegetables during breastfeeding: a randomized clinical trial of lactating mothers and infants. Am J Clin Nutr 2017;106:67–76.
15 BeckermanJP, Slade E, Ventura AK: Maternal diet during lactation and breast-feeding practices have synergistic association with child diet at 6 years. Public Health Nutr 2020;23:286–294.
16 George GC, Hanss-Nuss H, Milani TJ, Freeland-Graves JH: Food choices of low-income women during pregnancy and postpartum. J Am Diet Assoc 2005;105:899–907.

17 Anstey EH, Chen J, Elam-Evans LD, Perrine CG: Racial and geographic differences in breastfeeding – United States, 2011–2015. MMWR Morb Mortal Wkly Rep 2017;14;66:723–727.

18 Schindler-Ruwisch J, Roess A, Robert RC, Napolitano M: Limitations of workplace lactation support: the case for DC WIC recipients. J Hum Lact 2020;36:59–63.

19 Patnode CD, Henninger ML, Senger CA, et al: Primary care interventions to support breastfeeding: updated evidence report and systematic review for the US Preventive Services Task Force. JAMA 2016;316:1694–1705.

20 Campoy C, Campos D, Cerdo T, et al: Complementary feeding in developed countries: the 3 Ws (When, What, and Why?). Ann Nutr Metab 2018; 73:27–36.

21 Caton SJ, Ahern SM, Remy E, et al: Repetition counts: repeated exposure increases intake of a novel vegetable in UK pre-school children compared to flavour–flavour and flavour–nutrient learning. Br J Nutr 2013;109:2089–2097.

22 Barends C, de Vries JH, Mojet J, de Graaf C: Effects of starting weaning exclusively with vegetables on vegetable intake at the age of 12 and 23 months. Appetite 2014;81:193–199.

23 Coulthard H, Harris G, Fogel A: Exposure to vegetable variety in infants weaned at different ages. Appetite 2014;78:89–94.

24 Nucci AM, Virtanen SM, Sorkio S, et al: Regional differences in milk and complementary feeding patterns in infants participating in an international nutritional type 1 diabetes prevention trial. Matern Child Nutr 2017;13:e12354.

25 Moding KJ, Ferrante MJ, Bellows LL, et al: Variety and content of commercial infant and toddler vegetable products manufactured and sold in the United States. Am J Clin Nutr 2018;107:576–583.

26 Johnson SL: Developmental and environmental influences on young children's vegetable preferences and consumption. Adv Nutr 2016;7:220S–231S.

27 Fries LR, Martin N, van der Horst K: Parent-child mealtime interactions associated with toddlers' refusals of novel and familiar foods. Physiol Behav 2017;176:93–100.

28 Remington A, Anez E, Croker H, et al: Increasing food acceptance in the home setting: a randomized controlled trial of parent-administered taste exposure with incentives. Am J Clin Nutr 2012; 95:72–77.

29 Edelson LR, Mokdad C, Martin N: Prompts to eat novel and familiar fruits and vegetables in families with 1–3 year-old children: relationships with food acceptance and intake. Appetite 2016;99: 138–148.

30 Weinfield NS, Borger C, Au LE, et al: Longer participation in WIC is associated with better diet quality in 24-month-old children. J Acad Nutr Diet 2020;120:963–971.

Published online: November 12, 2020

Black MM, Singhal A, Hillman CH (eds): Building Future Health and Well-Being of Thriving Toddlers and Young Children. Nestlé Nutr Inst Workshop Ser. Basel, Karger, 2020, vol 95, pp 88–99 (DOI: 10.1159/000511515)

Introducing Hard-to-Like Foods to Infants and Toddlers: Mothers' Perspectives and Children's Experiences about Learning to Accept Novel Foods

Susan L. Johnson[a] Kameron J. Moding[b]

[a]Children's Eating Laboratory, Department of Pediatrics, Section of Nutrition, University of Colorado Anschutz Medical Campus, Aurora, CO, USA; [b]Department of Human Development and Family Studies, Purdue University, West Lafayette, IN, USA

Abstract

Children reportedly consume a variety of adequate vegetables during the introduction of complementary foods, and breastfeeding helps to facilitate child food acceptance. However, dietary intake of vegetables is reported to fall when children begin to eat foods of the family table. In laboratory settings, repeated exposure is effective in promoting children's acceptance and consumption of novel foods. We have recently explored mother and child early experiences (from infancy to toddlerhood) with offering hard-to-like foods. Our findings suggest a "sweet spot" for food introduction and acceptance during the early complementary feeding period (6–12 months) with increasing variability in acceptance and negative child behaviors occurring during toddlerhood. When queried, most mothers are familiar with repeated exposure concepts, but their persistence in continuing to offer disliked foods differs. Some report they will "never give up" – a stance linked to health beliefs and that children should "eat what we eat." Others seem more influenced by children's resistance and food dislikes, and the amounts their child eat. The majority believe that children's tastes change and that their child will accept rejected foods later. These mothers may reoffer a rejected food after "a break." Opportunities exist to translate repeated exposure paradigms to practical methods mothers can successfully adopt in the home.

Introduction

Some foods appear to be easier to like than others, and numerous influences take part to shape children's food preferences and acceptance patterns. These influences include hardwired, genetic reactions to basic tastants, exposure to flavors through maternal influences, the natural course of children's eating development, and family level influences. Children must learn to like foods, and which foods become accepted varies according to children's opportunities, and the quality of said opportunities for interaction with foods and flavors.

Often the foods that are most difficult to engage children to eat are the foods, like vegetables, that we most desire children to eat. Instilling children with a preference for these nutritious foods is vital for the development of healthy eating habits which, when carried through for a lifetime, are thought to reduce the risk of preventable chronic diseases [1]. Children's early experiences with such foods, via repeated exposures which caregivers utilize to acquaint children with these foods, tips the balance towards or away from their acceptance. Thus, the complementary feeding period is viewed as a critical developmental period for establishing eating behaviors and food acceptance patterns that can last a lifetime [2].

Emergence of Children's Food Preferences

Children are born with genetic predispositions to like certain tastes; sweetness is preferred at birth and even elicits responses in utero by the 2nd trimester [3]. Sweet tasting substances evoke positive facial reflexes associated with and interpreted as pleasure. This innate preference for sweetness is theorized to facilitate the consumption of foods that are safe, energy dense, and sometimes (as in the case of fruits) good sources of nutrients required for healthy growth. Other basic tastants, like bitterness and sourness, elicit negative facial reflexes like gapes, grimaces, and pursing of the lips. It should be noted, however, that these negative responses do not necessarily inhibit ingestion early in life [4].

Influences on children's food preferences start early in life, beginning in utero through transmission of flavors from the maternal diet into amniotic fluid [4]. For the infant who consumes human milk, the experience of receiving flavor exposure continues as, again, aromatic compounds from the maternal diet are transmitted to infants through breastfeeding, a veritable smorgasbord of flavor. Such flavor exposures have been noted to facilitate the transition to solid foods during complementary feeding and, later, to foods of the family table [3, 5, 6].

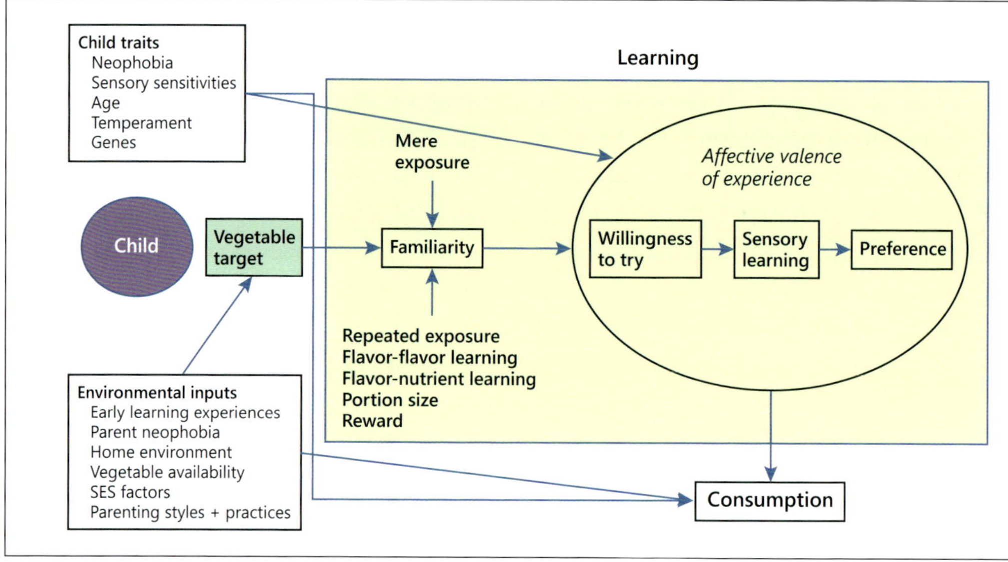

Fig. 1. A 2-stage model of influences on the development of children's vegetable preferences and consumption. Stage 1 reflects influences on children's willingness to try vegetables. Stage 2 considers inputs on children's vegetable consumption. SES, socioeconomic status. Original figure from Johnson [36].

Early and repeated experiences with flavor are thought to positively influence infants to more readily accept foods offered during the complementary feeding period, beginning around 6 months of age [6–9]. Sullivan and Birch [7] reported that infants who had been breastfed more readily accepted a novel vegetable as a first food than did infants with a history of formula feeding. Further, infants exposed to bitter tastes in protein hydrolysate formula more readily accepted and consumed such formula, and the effects of early exposure to these flavors persisted into the preschool years [8, 10].

These "natural experiments" of flavor transmission demonstrate the effects of repeated flavor exposure on children's acquisition of food acceptance patterns. Experimental studies employing repeated exposure have consistently confirmed that repetition, and the associative conditioning that occurs with exposure, are reliable paths towards increasing children's preference and consumption of initially disliked or rejected flavors [11, 12]. While most of these studies demonstrate short-term increases in children's preference and consumption, one longitudinal study has reported lasting effects of repeated exposure to both a target vegetable and vegetable variety on 6-year-old children's intake of a target vegetable [13].

Zajonc's [14] mere exposure theory, applied to food and eating, is the theoretical basis for these findings and posits that repeated positive interactions and experiences with novelty (whether food, music, or any other experience) result in familiarization and ultimate liking and acceptance. In the case of eating, exposure to novel foods and positive experiences with initially rejected foods leads to willingness to try the food and eventual consumption (Fig. 1). Multiple feeding trials conducted with infants and young children validate this theory, with younger infants responding more favorably than toddlers and preschoolers [10, 12]. One critical point is that repeated exposure increases *willingness to try* a target food before increases in *consumption* – a point often lost on caregivers who are more focused on increasing *how much* children eat of a given food [15].

Another potential influence on young children's emerging food preferences is proposed to occur when flavors of liked foods are mixed with flavors of less liked or disliked foods: the principle of associative conditioning of a flavor preference. A number of studies have paired known (milk) [12] or liked (peaches) [11] foods with vegetables and report improvements in consumption of the paired vegetables, and in the case of pairing with a sweet food, reductions in facial reactions of distaste. While improvements in infants' acceptance occurred, it is difficult to disentangle the effects of associative conditioning of flavors from repeated exposure effects given that multiple exposures occurred alongside the pairings of target foods with liked flavors, and no mere exposure condition was included in study designs. That said, the appearance of blends of fruit and vegetable in commercially prepared infant foods has reinforced these findings for consumers [16].

Developmental Influences on Children's Food Acceptance

Anatomical [17] and social-emotional aspects of children's development occur during infancy and toddlerhood which are associated with children's development of eating behavior [9, 18–21]. Maturation of the oral motor cavity, with increasing capacity to consume and manipulate semisolid and solid boluses, occurs during the period of 4–6 months of age, and the first teeth begin to appear around 6–8 months of age. Teething both positively and negatively influences children's food acceptance by (1) promoting the acceptance of more textured foods and (2) creating day-to-day challenges in children's appetites and responses to eating. Children also begin to gain more volitional control in eating as they advance towards toddlerhood. Gross and fine motor milestones (e.g., palmar and pincer grasps) emerge during this period of child development coinciding with children's desire and ability to begin self-feeding. During the complementary feeding period and on into toddlerhood, children's receptive and expressive language increases quickly, and, when motivated, children can follow simple directions and learn names of objects. During toddlerhood, food neophobia, or fear of new foods, and food jags also begin to occur; the toddler's growing desire for autonomy can be expressed as food refusal and negatively affect feeding [22]. Concurrently, children's energy needs for growth begin to slow, and the nexus of reduction in appetite, burgeoning food refusal, increased motoric capacity, and demands for autonomy can translate into heightened parental concern and confusion [9]. Feeding the toddler multiple times per day for meals and snacks can be a demanding, unrelenting parental role.

For infants and toddlers, such experiences may provide opportunities to continue to develop self-regulation in response to novelty. Repeated exposure to aversive stimuli could contribute to a toddler's ability to engage in a novel experience and may also facilitate the development of emotional aspects of self-regulation during eating [19, 23]. Responsive parenting and feeding help promote the development of emotional, social, and cognitive development, and help young children learn self-regulation of eating [23, 24].

Caregiver Influences on Children's Emerging Self-Regulation

Self-regulation is a complex construct that involves the capacity to regulate behaviors, cognitions, and emotions in the context of positive and negative situations. Self-regulation encompasses a broad array of processes, some of which relate to the development of eating behavior [25]. These processes include, but are not limited to, executive functioning, emotion regulation, effortful and reactive control, impulsivity, and delay of gratification [26].

Emotion regulation, one facet of children's self-regulation, develops over the second and third years, and is related to changes in children's growing cognitive and language abilities [25]. Spinrad et al. [27] suggested that caregiver responses to children's positive and negative affect influence children's budding emotional competence. Mothers' reactions to situations which their children find to be challenging can contribute to socializing children's emotional responses; positive or supporting responses help children to learn ways to regulate their states of arousal. Other maternal responses, e.g., giving in to their children's demands when children react negatively, may prevent children from developing strategies to cope with negative arousal or even lead to escalation of negative arousal [25].

In a longitudinal study, Spinrad et al. [27] reported that mothers more often responded to 18-month-old children's negative affect (compared to positive affect); some using distraction, some giving in to the child's wishes, and others questioning the validity of the child's emotions (e.g., "why are you crying?"). At 30 months, these kinds of maternal responses were used less frequently, and the use of verbal explanation increased. Thus, as children's cognitive and language abilities increased, mothers used more verbal explanations or reasoning. Of note, when mothers "gave in" and granted children's wishes, or questioned the validity of their reactions when children were 18 months of age, their children continued to display greater negative affect (and lower emotional self-regulation) in response to disappointment at 30 months of age. These researchers suggest that when children are indulged during challenging moments, they are also denied opportunities to learn self-regulation for similar future challenges.

Neophobia Emergence and Challenges

Applied to the child feeding context, we pose that caregiver responses to children's negative reactions to a novel food could invoke the same pattern of interactions between children and their caregivers. For example, when children are introduced to a food that is disliked, and they exhibit negative affect, and consequently the caregiver withdraws that food and replaces it with a better-accepted food (in the name of getting the child to eat enough), the child's rejecting behavior is reinforced by the offering of a more-preferred food. This scenario represents one pathway by which picky eating could emerge and be unintentionally reinforced. Alternatively, when children's negative reactions are met with equanimity, and the food continues to be offered but expectations of consumption are limited, this offers an opportunity to the child to become familiar with the food and to learn to regulate their reactions to experiences with novel foods.

In the Good Tastes Study, infants showed variability in their response to the taste of a bitter, novel vegetable, with some infants avidly accepting the food and others grimacing, gaping, and crying in response to the taste (Fig. 2) [28]. However, negative responses did not result in the youngest infants (<12 months of age) refusing to accept another taste of the same vegetable. That children responded negatively but continued to accept the next bite suggests that young infants may respond reflexively to the visual cue of a spoon loaded with food coming towards them: opening their mouths to accept the bite. Toddlers (between 12 and 24 months of age) in the Good Tastes Study exhibited greater reactivity to the taste of the food, and those who showed negative reactions were more likely to reject subsequent offers.

Previously, it has been noted that infants who are breastfed receive exposure to a greater variety of flavors than infants who are formula fed, and these flavor experiences confer an advantage for the breastfed infant in accepting first foods.

stead of indicating absolute rejection, these could be reflexive responses to novel tastes [3]. It may be appropriate to encourage mothers to persist in the face of initial negative facial responses and spitting out of foods that are unfamiliar if these responses stop short of children crying, gagging, or showing strong displeasure.

Mothers' stated feeding priorities included getting children to eat (enough), good nutrition, and exposure to a healthy diet, the child's satisfaction both with specific foods served at an eating occasion and a good relationship with food generally, satisfying the child's energy needs and avoiding mood swings associated with hunger, and promoting children's acceptance of a wide variety of foods from different cultures, thus preventing their children from becoming picky eaters.

Our findings echo those of Carruth et al. [31] published in 1998, who reported decades ago that mothers' intentions to re-offer rejected foods varies widely. While more mothers in the recent study indicated that they would re-offer a food a sufficient number of exposures to facilitate acceptance, the time period over which they would do so also varied from days, to months, and even years. A gap in knowledge regarding repeated exposure methods is illuminated by these findings: the optimal interval across which exposures can be offered has not been explored fully by researchers and varies dramatically in caregiver practice. Further, more research is necessary to determine whether early acceptance (during complementary feeding) is associated with reductions in picky eating or food neophobia.

When asked about their emotions and reactions when their children rejected a food, most mothers from our survey reported they were surprisingly indifferent. Of those who stated frustration or sadness, these emotions were most often related to wastes of time, money, and food, or that their child would miss out on the healthfulness of the food rather than disappointment that the child had not enjoyed the food.

Caregiver Feeding Priorities and the Influence on Maternal Persistence in Offering Difficult-to-Like Foods

From the findings of our survey, as well as those of previous studies [32], what emerges is that mothers have competing priorities for feeding their young infants and toddlers. Goals for nutrition, health, and eating collide with concerns about whether their child is eating enough [33, 34] to sustain optimal growth and development. Ultimately, what appears to count most for mothers is how much children consume, and how easily this happens during feeding [6], ensuring that their children enjoy eating. Mothers attend to children's facial responses to foods in the early complementary feeding period, and what seems, understandably, to dictate mothers' responses is how difficult it is to accomplish the end goal of getting their child to eat. By the time children reach toddlerhood, feeding challenges often escalate, and the multiple-times-per-day task of feeding their child, who is increasingly demanding autonomy (though not necessarily ready for it), can become less and less rewarding. Thus, persisting to offer foods that may rate highly for nutrition and health, but that make the feeding and parenting experience consistently onerous, can be a tall order, whereas alternative strategies like "taking a break" from the food or coercive and pressuring feeding practices may yield better short-term outcomes for how much children consume [20].

Conclusions

It would seem that future research would best be oriented towards methods to help caregivers learn to persist in offering difficult-to-like foods until they reap the rewards of children's acceptance of these foods, instilling confidence and trust in the process of repeated exposure and the concept that children generally will eat enough to meet their energy needs when offered a balanced, nutritious diet. Additional studies should be undertaken to determine whether taking "breaks" in offering previously rejected foods improves or detracts from building liking, and to determine whether an optimal interval exists during which exposures should take place to build lasting improvements in acceptance for difficult-to-like foods.

Caregivers desire information and strategies to help their children participate in family meals and to learn to have a healthful relationship with food and eating [35]. Promoting children's autonomy and their development of self-regulation skills may help with challenging mealtimes during the toddler period.

Acknowledgments

We would like to acknowledge the efforts of Haley Lucitt, MSPH, who designed and administered the Good Tastes Survey.

Conflict of Interest Statement

The work presented herein was funded by an investigator-initiated research grant from the Sugar Association. Both authors received salary and research support from this grant. The funder has not participated in, nor been privy to, study design, data analyses, or the writing of this publication. The authors have no additional conflicts to report.

References

1 Schulze MB, Martínez-González MA, Fung TT, et al: Food based dietary patterns and chronic disease prevention. BMJ 2018;361:k2396.
2 Craigie AM, Lake AA, Kelly SA, et al: Tracking of obesity-related behaviours from childhood to adulthood: a systematic review. Maturitas 2011; 70:266–284.
3 Nicklaus S: 13 – Relationships between early flavor exposure, and food acceptability and neophobia; in Etiévant P, Guichard E, Salles C, Voilley A (eds): Flavor: From Food to Behaviors, Wellbeing and Health. Duxford, Woodhead Publishing, 2016, pp 293–311.
4 Mennella JA, Nicklaus S, Jagolino AL, Yourshaw LM: Variety is the spice of life: strategies for promoting fruit and vegetable acceptance during infancy. Physiol Behav 2008;94:29–38.
5 Hausner H, Nicklaus S, Issanchou S, et al: Breastfeeding facilitates acceptance of a novel dietary flavour compound. e-SPEN 2009;4:e231–e238.
6 Gerrish CJ, Mennella JA: Flavor variety enhances food acceptance in formula-fed infants. Am J Clin Nutr 2001;73:1080–1085.
7 Sullivan SA, Birch LL: Infant dietary experience and acceptance of solid foods. Pediatrics 1994;93: 271–277.
8 Mennella JA, Griffin CE, Beauchamp GK: Flavor programming during infancy. Pediatrics 2004; 113:840–845.
9 Schwartz C, Vandenberghe-Descamps M, Sulmont-Rossé C, et al: Behavioral and physiological determinants of food choice and consumption at sensitive periods of the life span, a focus on infants and elderly. Innov Food Sci Emerg Technol 2018;46:91–106.
10 Anzman-Frasca S, Ehrenberg S: Learning to like: roles of repeated exposure and other types of learning; in Lumeng JC, Fisher JO (eds): Pediatric Food Preferences and Eating Behaviors. London, Academic Press, 2018, pp 35–52.
11 Forestell CA, Mennella JA: Early determinants of fruit and vegetable acceptance. Pediatrics 2007; 120:1247–1254.
12 Hetherington MM, Schwartz C, Madrelle J, et al: A step-by-step introduction to vegetables at the beginning of complementary feeding. The effects of early and repeated exposure. Appetite 2015;84: 280–290.
13 Maier-Nöth A, Schaal B, Leathwood P, Issanchou S: The lasting influences of early food-related variety experience: a longitudinal study of vegetable acceptance from 5 months to 6 years in two populations. PLoS One 2016;11:e0151356.
14 Zajonc RB: Attitudinal effects of mere exposure. J Pers Soc Psychol 1968;9:1.
15 Johnson SL, Ryan SM, Kroehl M, et al: A longitudinal intervention to improve young children's liking and consumption of new foods: findings from the Colorado LEAP study. Int J Behav Nutr Phys Act 2019;16:49.
16 Moding KJ, Ferrante MJ, Bellows LL, et al: Variety and content of commercial infant and toddler vegetable products manufactured and sold in the United States. Am J Clin Nutr 2018;107:576–583.
17 Gee BM, Engle J, Parker C, et al: Frequency and duration of developmental fine motor patterns in infants and toddlers: a pilot cohort study. Ann Int Occup Ther 2019;3:21–28.
18 Johnson SL, Hayes JE: Developmental readiness, caregiver and child feeding behaviors, and sensory science as a framework for feeding young children. Nutr Today 2017;52(suppl):S30–S40.
19 Birch LL, Doub AE: Learning to eat: birth to age 2 years. Am J Clin Nutr 2014;99:723S–728S.
20 Cole NC, An R, Lee S-Y, Donovan SM: Correlates of picky eating and food neophobia in young children: a systematic review and meta-analysis. Nutr Rev 2017;75:516–532.
21 Carruth BR, Ziegler PJ, Gordon A, Hendricks K: Developmental milestones and self-feeding behaviors in infants and toddlers. J Am Diet Assoc 2004;104:51–56.
22 Johnson SL, Moding KJ, Bellows LL: Children's challenging eating behaviors: picky eating, food neophobia, and food selectivity; in Lumeng JC, Fisher JO (eds): Pediatric Food Preferences and Eating Behaviors. London, Academic Press, 2018, pp 73–92.

23 Stoeckel LE, Birch LL, Heatherton T, et al: Psychological and neural contributions to appetite self-regulation. Obesity 2017;25(S1):S17–S25.
24 Black MM, Aboud FE: Responsive feeding is embedded in a theoretical framework of responsive parenting. J Nutr 2011;141:490–494.
25 Kopp CB: Regulation of distress and negative emotions: a developmental view. Dev Psychol 1989;25:343.
26 Baker S, Morawska A, Mitchell A: Promoting children's healthy habits through self-regulation via parenting. Clin Child Family Psychol Rev 2019;22:52–62.
27 Spinrad TL, Stifter CA, Donelan-McCall N, Turner L: Mothers' regulation strategies in response to toddlers' affect: links to later emotion self-regulation. Soc Dev 2004;13:40–55.
28 Johnson S, Moding K, Hayes JE, et al: The Good Tastes Study: infants' and toddlers' acceptance of a familiar food and novel green bitter vegetable purees. American Society for Nutrition (ASN) Annual Meeting 2018.
29 Schwartz C, Issanchou S, Nicklaus S: Developmental changes in the acceptance of the five basic tastes in the first year of life. Br J Nutr 2009;102: 1375–1385.
30 Johnson S, Moding K, Flesher A, et al: The Good Tastes Study: relations between children's eating behaviors and caregivers' intentions to persist in offering difficult-to-like foods (OR03-02-19). Curr Dev Nutr 2019;3(suppl 1).
31 Carruth BR, Skinner J, Houck K, et al: The phenomenon of "picky eater": a behavioral marker in eating patterns of toddlers. J Am Coll Nutr 1998; 17:180–186.
32 Holley CE, Farrow C, Haycraft E: Investigating offering of vegetables by caregivers of preschool age children. Child Care Health Dev 2017;43: 240–249.
33 McNally J, Hugh-Jones S, Hetherington MM: "An invisible map" – maternal perceptions of hunger, satiation and "enough" in the context of baby led and traditional complementary feeding practices. Appetite 2020;148:104608.
34 Spill MK, Callahan EH, Shapiro MJ, et al: Caregiver feeding practices and child weight outcomes: a systematic review. Am J Clin Nutr 2019; 109(suppl 7):990S–1002S.
35 Hepworth A, Brick T, Small M: Exploring parents' satisfaction with infant and toddler feeding information: a repeated-measures analysis of information need and acquisition characteristics (P17-006-19). Curr Dev Nutr 2019;3(suppl 1):nzz038.P17-006-19.
36 Johnson SL: Developmental and environmental influences on young children's vegetable preferences and consumption. Adv Nutr 2016;7:220S–231S.

Published online: November 9, 2020
Black MM, Singhal A, Hillman CH (eds): Building Future Health and Well-Being of Thriving Toddlers and Young Children. Nestlé Nutr Inst Workshop Ser. Basel, Karger, 2020, vol 95, pp 100–111 (DOI: 10.1159/000511524)

Dietary Sugars: Not as Sour as They Are Made Out to Be

Dennis M. Bier
Department of Pediatrics, Children's Nutrition Research Center, Baylor College of Medicine, Houston, TX, USA

Abstract

Over the course of evolution, Mother Nature preserved the ability of humans to make every sugar they need for metabolic functions. Glucose is the almost exclusive fuel preferred by the human brain. Human infants are born with sweet taste receptors, sugars are a significant energy source in human milk, and mammals have a direct gut-to-brain sugar-sensing system that enhances development of a preference for sugars. If sugars are as toxic as many postulate, what species advantage was conferred by this evolutionary progression? Observational studies have reported that sugar consumption is associated with various adverse health risks. However, observational studies can never prove causality, dietary intake records are known to be highly problematic, and the huge number of correlation interdependencies among environmental "exposome" variables makes it impossible to attribute causality to individual dietary components. Additionally, these studies overall have been graded as low quality, and many reported the small effect sizes are likely within the propagated methodological "noise." With several exceptions, data from randomized controlled trials that ensured isocaloric energy intakes have failed to confirm the causal implications of the observational data. Likewise, the comprehensive UK Scientific Committee on Nutrition Report on Carbohydrates and Health also failed to confirm the vast majority of widely postulated detrimental effects of sugar consumption per se. Current data on intakes of sugar-sweetened beverages and on the risks associated with high intakes of dietary fructose remain under debate.

Historical Background

For more than 50 years, nutritionists and physicians have debated the optimal macronutrient composition of one's diet that will promote health and minimize the risk of developing chronic diseases. Over time, the pendulum has swung from higher/lower percentages of dietary fats to higher/lower percentages of dietary carbohydrates (for one cannot change one without correspondingly changing the other in the opposite direction, if one wants to maintain energy balance) and back again. At present, prevailing opinions place fats in the ascendency and carbohydrates in the descendancy.

Over the approximately 6 million years of human evolution, our species has evolved the metabolic "machinery" to live well on whatever local macronutrients are available in sufficient amounts to supply our biological needs. Thus, we are omnivores, and the individual members of our species consume varying diets of diverse composition worldwide. Some diets are very dependent on carbohydrates as their primary source of energy. Others are principally dependent on fats to supply energy. Despite these very wide differences, when one excludes obvious reasons for accelerated mortality like wars, famines, and the like, humans tend to live similar, relatively long lives irrespective of their differences in macronutrient intakes. For sure, there are differences in the lifespan that can be associated with components of the human diet [1]. The implication of the associations is, of course, that they reflect causality. Nonetheless, given the inadequacy of the methods to determine actual food intakes and the innumerable, unmeasured, unaccounted for environmental variables that constitute covarying interdependencies present within our vast "exosome," it is impossible to calculate confidently which and/or how much of the risk differences are due to diets alone or to the macronutrient contents of those diets. In fact, it is difficult to know for sure if any of the differences are due to diet alone. Nonetheless, this has not prevented expert groups from trying [1] although the nonlinear nature of the associations further compounds the difficulty and confounds the conclusions [2]. Recognizing these limitations, in western societies reflected by the UK, the lowest all-cause mortality risks appear to be associated with dietary intakes of about 40–55% energy from carbohydrates and on the order of 30–40% energy from dietary fats [3]; good news since, overall, these are the ranges in most commonly consumed western diets. Now, as difficult as it is to ascribe causal long-term risk conclusions to dietary macronutrients, the discussion following will attempt to focus on the constituent components of one of the macronutrient classes, dietary sugars. Needless to say, related discussion about individual fats constituting dietary fat intakes is also taking place elsewhere [4].

Axioms

Before doing so, however, it is critical to lay out the axioms underlying the theorem under development. First, sugars are not, per se, defined as dietary essential nutrients in the traditional nutrition sense since the human body can make every sugar it needs. In fact, I might use the latter observation as an argument that Mother Nature considers sugars as the truly essential nutrients because She did not leave their adequate internal supply to the vagaries of the available external food supply.

Furthermore, in directly related sense, dietary sugars do contain the essential external nutrient, energy, a critical essential nutrient for sustaining human life in many societies worldwide. However, relatively recently, consumption of excess energy has been a leading contribution to the development of human obesity worldwide. So, the first axiom in my thesis below is that sugars should not be consumed in amounts that contribute to excess energy intake. This axiom applies to dietary fat or protein intakes as well since they, too, are sources of energy. In fact, dietary fats contribute considerably more energy per gram than dietary sugars. For example, Mozaffarian et al. [5] showed that increased consumption of red and processed meat contributes as much, or more, to weight gain over a 4-year period than consumption of sugar-sweetened beverages (SSBs).

The second axiom for agreement a priori is that the consumption of dietary sugars should not be in an amount that interferes with the consumption of the 40 or so essential dietary nutrients necessary to satisfy nutritional adequacy. No single food is an adequate source of all essential nutrients, and dietary sugars should not be consumed in quantities that reduce intakes of the variety of foods necessary to establish and maintain nutritional sufficiency. Although the fraction of dietary energy contributed by sugars in some individuals in western societies now appears to approach the level necessary to convey this risk, the amount of sugars consumed by most people still does not. Thus, given the 2 axiomatic conditions, the following exposition will focus on the risks of sugars per se on human health risks. In other words, I will focus on sugars themselves and not on human misuse of dietary sugar consumption. I do so because much of the literature either confuses the two, or because one direction of the literature argues aggressively for the fact that sugars per se are detrimental to humans.

Arguments from an Evolutionary Perspective

Table 1 summarizes various observations that support a thesis that human evolutionary development is inconsistent with the implication that sugars are toxic substances in themselves. Of course, no arguments of this kind prove causality,

Table 1. Has Mother Nature tried to fool us for millions of years?

1.	Humans can synthesize every sugar necessary for life; from Mother Nature's perspective, sugars are the most essential macronutrients
2.	Glucose is the only important fuel for the human fetus
3.	Infants are born with sweet taste receptors, and about one-third of human milk energy is supplied by sugar
4.	Humans are born with a gut-to-brain sugar-sensing pathway that promotes development of a behavioral preference for sugar
5.	Glucose is the only fuel preferred by the brain, resulting in irreversible oxidation of the majority of glucose produced daily by the liver; in the absence of an external supply of new carbon for gluconeogenesis, the body breaks down muscle protein amino acids to replenish glucose carbon necessary to maintain brain oxidative energy needs

but taken together they provide a strong body of evidence that speaks against a proposition that sugars are toxic substances in their own right. First, as mentioned above, humans can synthesize every sugar they need while they must obtain 2 fatty acids and 8 or 9 amino acids from external dietary sources. It would appear entirely counterintuitive that evolutionary progression would proceed in this direction if sugars were toxic per se. Secondly, glucose is the only significant fuel for the mammalian fetus. This fact has been established conclusively by decades of experimental studies and clinical observations. Moreover, there are specific placental glucose transporters and other fetoplacental substrate metabolic exchange mechanisms that optimize the delivery of glucose to the fetus. It defies credulity that evolution of the mammalian species progressed in a manner that established glucose as the principal, almost exclusive, fetal fuel and simultaneously developed fetoplacental mechanisms to ensure an adequate fetal glucose supply were glucose is a toxic substance.

It is well established that human infants are born with sweet taste receptors. One must seriously consider why this would be an evolutionary advantage if developing a taste for sweetness was detrimental to infant survival, health, and development. Furthermore, the sugar content of human milk is considerably higher than that of other mammalian species. Approximately one-third of the energy supplied by human milk comes from the disaccharide lactose. One must again question the evolutionary advantage of progression to a species milk supply high in sugar if, in fact, the sugar was detrimental to the species. Even more importantly, mammals are born with a sugar-sensing system in the gut that "speaks" directly to the brain, promoting a behavioral, developmental pathway for sugar preference [6]. What possible species advantage is conferred by evolving such a mechanism if the end result proved toxic to the species?

Finally, the human brain prefers, almost exclusively, glucose as the fuel for its activities. The brain consumes and oxidizes approximately two-thirds of the glucose produced daily by the liver. I believe that few would argue with the "philosophical" thesis that the human brain represents the highest evolutionary achievement in biology as we know it. If so, what is a possible, even remotely plausible, reason for the brain's choice of a simple sugar as its preferred (almost only) source of fuel for its activities, if this sugar, itself, were a toxic substance? Additionally, in the context of dietary sugar consumption, we must consider the following mass balance issue. Brain glucose oxidation results in irreversible conversion of glucose carbon to expired carbon dioxide. In other words, net glucose carbon leaves the body forever. This is no trivial loss of carbon given the fact that the brain oxidizes the majority of glucose produced daily by the liver. Although the liver can make new glucose via gluconeogenesis, the only new internal carbons for net new glucose synthesis come from amino acid carbons stored as muscle proteins. Carbons made into glucose via the Cori cycle are carbons recycled via lactate and pyruvate. As such, they are not new carbons and cannot replace carbons irreversibly lost via CO_2. For this reason, if there is no dietary source of glucose or of gluconeogenic carbons available from other ingested macronutrients, the body must break down muscle protein to feed the brain. Depending on age or feeding state, this carbon requirement can amount to >100 g of "glucose equivalents" daily. This is clearly not a desirable circumstance over the long term. In the only controlled human experiment of its kind of which I am aware [7], we know that the need for external carbon sources to make new glucose fuel for the brain is eventually reduced by reduction in brain energy needs and by ketone body replacement for glucose as the fuel source for the brain.

Arguments from the Perspective of Metabolism in Childhood

Forty to 50 years ago, there was a concerted effort among pediatric endocrinologists to find a means of identifying in families having a child with type 1 diabetes other children in the same family who might be at increased risk for future development of diabetes. For this reason, the oral glucose tolerance tests (OGTTs) were performed in hundreds of children at a time when most children were lean. Unfortunately, most of these data have vanished from the present view. The standard test dose was 1.75 g of glucose per kilogram ideal body weight up to a maximum dose of 100 g of glucose. A 12-oz can of soda contains about 40 g of sugar, approximately half as glucose and half as fructose. Since fructose has essentially no effect on the postingestion circulating glucose level, the maxi-

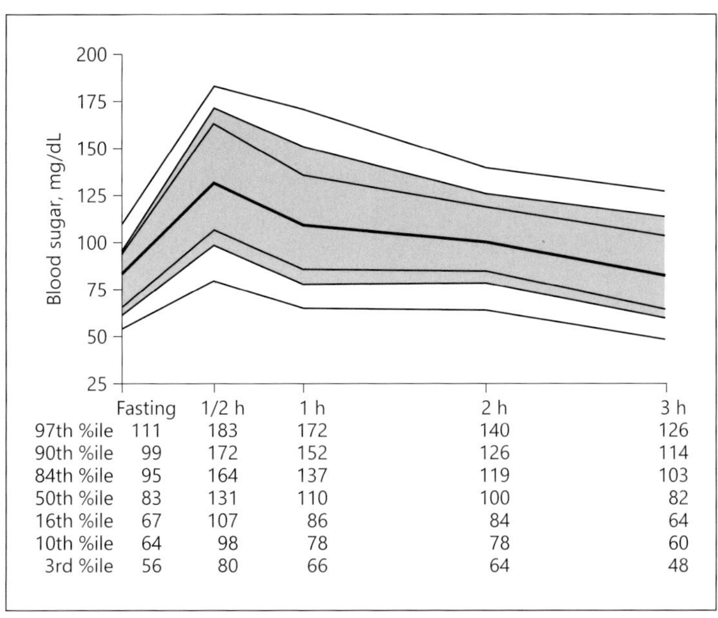

	Fasting	1/2 h	1 h	2 h	3 h
97th %ile	111	183	172	140	126
90th %ile	99	172	152	126	114
84th %ile	95	164	137	119	103
50th %ile	83	131	110	100	82
16th %ile	67	107	86	84	64
10th %ile	64	98	78	78	60
3rd %ile	56	80	66	64	48

Fig. 1. Blood glucose values in 200 normal children during a standard oral glucose tolerance test [8].

mum glucose dose during an OGTT is equivalent to the glucose dose in about 5 cans of soda. Despite the magnitude of the oral glucose load during an OGTT, approximately 10% of children show no clear peak circulating glucose level above the fasting level in the hours immediately following glucose ingestion. In other words, the insulin secretory capacity and the peripheral insulin sensitivity in these children are such that they are able to dispose of an oral glucose dose very rapidly without any clearly discernable rise in the circulating glucose level. In OGTTs carried out in 200 children by Guthrie et al. [8], 50% of the children had blood glucose levels <131 mg/dL 30 min after glucose ingestion, and 50% had blood glucose levels <110 mg/dL 1 h after consumption of the glucose dose (Fig. 1) [8]. Knopf et al. [9] performed OGGTs in 100 children and found almost identical results. In this case, the vast majority of children had a blood glucose level <120 mg/dL by 60 min after ingestion, when the mean blood glucose level was approximately 100 mg/dL, not much higher than the fasting blood glucose value. In other words, healthy lean children have a very high capacity to deal with a glucose load.

Nearly 2 decades ago, Sunehag et al. [10–12] and Treuth et al. [13] engaged in a series of studies confirming that lean children and adolescents were capable of dealing rapidly to alterations in dietary macronutrient content. The group conducted a series of dietary studies in which the subjects consumed isocaloric, isonitrogenous diets for 7 days that were either high in fat (55% energy) or high in carbohydrates (60% energy). As such, to maintain a constant energy intake, both diets correspondingly contained 30% energy from carbohydrates or 25% energy from fat, respectively [10–14]. In some of the subjects, the dietary carbohydrate content was constituted so that fructose was responsible for 6 or 24% of dietary energy [12]. The subjects' energy balance was assessed using room respiration calorimetry, the proportion of macronutrient fuels oxidized was calculated from the respiratory quotient, glucose production rates, gluconeogenic rates, and lipolytic rates were quantified from stable, isotopically labeled substrate infusions, insulin secretory dynamics and insulin sensitivity were measured using stable isotopically labeled intravenous or oral glucose tolerance tests with accepted minimal modeling approaches [10–14]. These studies showed clearly that healthy, lean children are fully capable of appropriately adjusting their energy expenditure and the proportions of dietary carbohydrate and/or fat oxidized to match wide changes in the macronutrient contents of their diets [13]. Substrate fuel kinetics were minimally affected [10]. Because of their high levels of insulin sensitivity, prepubertal children were able to adapt to a high carbohydrate intake with essentially no change in insulin secretion while adolescents did so with an appropriate increase in both insulin secretion and peripheral insulin sensitivity [10]. Dietary fructose content ranging from 6 to 24% energy intake has no effect on any of these parameters [10, 12, 13]. Again, healthy lean children are perfectly capable of adjusting their internal metabolic milieu and its regulatory "machinery" to accommodate wide changes in dietary macronutrient composition. Once a child becomes obese, however, his or her ability to improve insulin sensitivity when challenged with a high carbohydrate diet is impaired [11, 12]. Correspondingly, these obese individuals had to increase their insulin secretory rates more than twofold to maintain circulating glucose homeostasis [11, 12]. Nevertheless, ingestion of dietary fructose at intake levels responsible for 6–24% total energy (approximately 45–180 g fructose daily) had no effect on insulin secretion or insulin sensitivity (Fig. 2). Nor was there any effect on glucose kinetics or lipolysis. It is important to recognize here that the situation might be different in adults with established obesity since very carefully controlled SSB trials by Stanhope et al. [15, 16] were able to demonstrate that dietary fructose decreased insulin sensitivity in overweight/obese adults [15] and increased cardiovascular risk factors [15, 16], the latter not measured in the pediatric studies of Sunehag et al. [10–12, 14] and Treuth et al. [13]. Moreover, Stanhope and her colleagues from multiple academic institutions have recently provided a rationale for fructose as a causal agent in the development of hepatic insulin resistance [17].

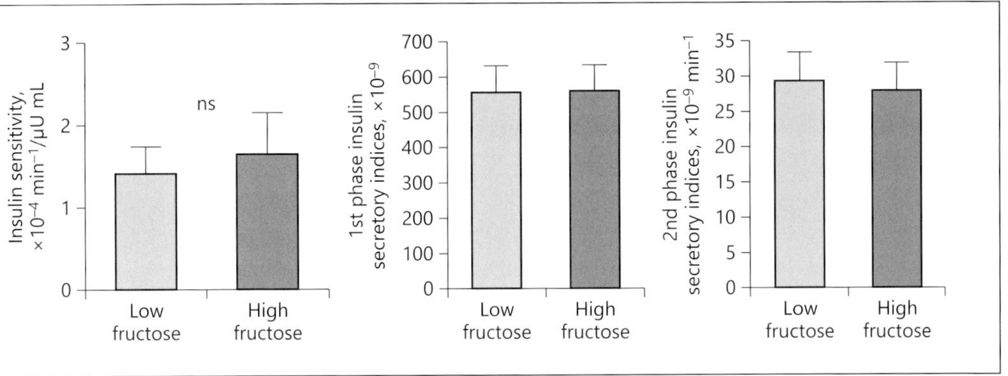

Fig. 2. Insulin secretory dynamics and insulin sensitivity measured following a stable-label intravenous glucose tolerance test in 6 adolescents who were studied before and after 7-day consumption of an isocaloric, isonitrogenous high-carbohydrate (60% energy) diet in which either 6 or 24% of dietary energy was supplied by fructose [13].

Arguments from the Perspective of Estimating Adult Chronic Disease Risks

Today, a significant fraction of criticism leveled at the consumption of dietary sugars focuses on the role of sugars as causative agents that increase adult chronic disease risk, particularly the risk for cardiovascular disease (CVD). Necessarily, most of the studies assessing these risks are observational in nature. In this context, it is critical to recognize the limitations of the methods widely used in such studies, and how they contribute to the confidence one can assign to the estimated increased relative risks, particularly to relative risk changes that are not much higher than 1.0 [18–20]. These limitations are widely ignored by authors who not only uncritically report small increases in relative risks, but also frequently use causal wording and/or imply causality when, in fact, an observational study can never prove causality, no matter how good or large it might be. For example, a recent observational study [21] on the risks of meat consumption reported that increased absolute all-cause mortality risks were <2% over a 30-year period but claimed that higher intakes of processed meat and unprocessed red meat were statistically associated with a 3–7% increase in incident CVD and all-cause mortality. Given the propagated known errors associated with food intake methods and food composition tables, and the uncertainties introduced by unmeasured unaccounted-for "exosome" confounders and their interdependencies, it is inconceivable that risk differences of this magnitude reflect detection of a true causal signal outside the level of methodological "noise" [21].

Table 2. UKSACN found no association of dietary sugar or sugar-sweetened beverage (SSB) intake with, or effect on, the following clinical or laboratory outcomes

Dietary sugar intake	SSB intake
Coronary events	BMI
Systolic blood pressure	Body fat
Total cholesterol	Colon cancer
LDL cholesterol	
Fasting triglycerides	
Fasting glucose	
Fasting insulin	
Risk of type 2 diabetes mellitus	

In 2015, the UK Scientific Advisory Committee on Nutrition (UKSACN) published its extensive report on carbohydrates and health [22]. This 384-page report was 9 years in the making, and its analyses were documented with 2,765 pages of supporting data. It is highly unlikely that another report as comprehensive as this one will be published anytime in the foreseeable future. Moreover, despite more recent additional publications on the relationships among dietary sugar intake and chronic disease risks, none of these, in my estimation, changes the findings of UKSACN. Tables 2–4 present a summary of the principal conclusions of the UKSACN report [22].

UKSACN found no association of dietary sugar intake with coronary events, blood pressure, total or LDL cholesterol, fasting triglycerides, fasting glucose or insulin, or the risk of type 2 diabetes mellitus (T2DM) (Table 2) [22], nor did it find a relationship of SSB intake and BMI, body fat, or colon cancer (Table 2) [22]. In cohort studies (Table 3), there was insufficient evidence to conclude that a relationship existed among mono- and disaccharide intakes and CVD events, or sugar-rich foods or SSB intakes and coronary events, blood pressure, body fat, fat distribution, and weight gain, or sugar-rich food consumption and T2DM, or SSB consumption and hypertension, energy intake, glycemia, insulinemia, and insulin sensitivity (Table 3) [22]. From reported randomized controlled trials (Table 4), there was insufficient evidence to conclude that relationships existed among sugar intake and vascular compliance, CRP, impaired glucose tolerance or HbA_{1C}, and caries in mixed/permanent teeth [22]. The report was also unable to conclude from randomized controlled trials that relationships existed among SSB intakes and fasting blood lipids, glycemia, insulinemia, insulin sensitivity, body weight, weight gain, and energy intake [22].

On the other hand, UKSACN was able to conclude that there were "fairly consistent" data showing that sugar intake can result in higher energy intakes,

Table 3. UKSACN found insufficient evidence in cohort studies to conclude that relationships existed between dietary sugar or sugar-sweetened beverage (SSB) intake and the following clinical and laboratory outcomes

Mono-/disaccharides and cardiovascular events	Sugar-rich foods and type 2 diabetes mellitus
Sugar-rich foods or SSB and coronary events	SSB and energy intake, glycemia, insulinemia, and insulin sensitivity
Sugar-rich foods and blood pressure	SSB and total or HDL cholesterol
SSB and hypertension	SSB and oral cancer
Sugar-rich foods or SSB on body fat, fat distribution, and weight gain	Frequency of SSB intake and caries in mixed and permanent teeth

Table 4. UKSACN found insufficient evidence in randomized controlled trials concluding that dietary sugars or sugar-sweetened beverage (SSB) intake caused the following clinical and laboratory outcomes

Sugar intake and vascular compliance	Sugar intake and impaired glucose tolerance or HbA_{1C}
Sugar intake and C-reactive protein	SSB intake and glycemia, insulinemia, or insulin sensitivity
Glucose, fructose, sucrose, or SSB and fasting blood lipids	SSB and periodontal disease
SSB and body weight, weight gain, and energy intake	Sugar-rich foods and caries in mixed/permanent teeth

even though this effect appeared to be the result of increased energy intake. Only 1 trial provided diets that were "designed to be iso-energetic and differ in the type of CHO provided." Moreover, this study was confounded by some subjects losing weight, some subjects gaining weight on lower energy intakes, and on "a spontaneous increase in energy intake on the high fat intervention relative to the three high carbohydrate interventions" [22]. Finally, although UKSACN concluded that an effect was demonstrated in observational studies "between sugar-sweetened beverage consumption and higher incidence of type 2 diabetes mellitus," confidence in this finding was weakened by the lack of association between sugar consumption and T2DM, the failure to demonstrate an association between SSB intake and BMI or body fat, and the inability to exclude confounding [22].

Naturally, additional studies have appeared in the literature since the publication of the UKSACN report 5 years ago. One of these [23], a systematic review and dose-response meta-analysis of 24 prospective cohort studies in 624,128 individuals, concluded that "current evidence supports a threshold of harm for intakes of total sugars, added sugars, and fructose at higher exposure and lack of harm for sucrose independent of form for CVD mortality" although the quality of evidence for that conclusion was low [23]. The thresholds for harm were 133 g of total sugars (26% energy), 58 g of fructose (11% energy), and 65 g of added sugars (13% energy). One must interpret these data cautiously. They failed to show a relationship among sugar intakes and the incidence of CVD, nor was an association found between added sugar intake and CVD mortality across the whole dietary intake range. Paradoxically, sucrose intake was associated with decreased CVD mortality risk [23]. Moreover, the increased relative risk of CVD mortality was on the order of 8–9%, a change likely within the propagated "noise level" of observational methods [23]. A related analysis [24] was unable to find an association among total sugars or fructose intakes and T2DM while sucrose intake, again, was associated with a decreased risk of T2DM. Finally, in 6 cohorts totaling 240,506 subjects, every additional SSB consumed from none to ≥1 daily increased the incident hypertension risk by 8.2% [25].

Conclusion

It is almost impossible today to read an article, either in the nutritional literature or in the public media, that does not conclude that dietary sugars are harmful. However, there are a series of arguments based on evolutionary preservation of favorable traits, the ability of lean individuals, particularly nonobese children, to readily metabolize dietary sugars, and the limited degree of confidence to which one can ascribe causal implications from observational studies reporting small changes in relative risks that should give one pause in believing that sugars in the diet are as sour as they are commonly made out to be.

Conflict of Interest Statement

In the last 3 years, Dr. Bier has received consultant and/or lecture fees and/or reimbursements for travel, hotel, and other expenses from the International Life Sciences Institute; the International Council on Amino Acid Science; Nutrition, and Growth Solutions, Inc.; Ajinomoto, Co.; the Lorenzini Foundation; the Nutrition Coalition, the CrossFit Foundation; the International Glutamate Technical Committee; Nestlé S.A.; Ferrero SpA; Indiana University; the National Institutes of Health; Mallinckrodt Pharmaceuticals; the Infant Nutrition Council of America; and the Israel Institute.

References

1 GBD 2017 Diet Collaborators: Health effects of dietary risks in 195 countries, 1990–2017: a systematic analysis for the Global Burden of Disease Study 2017. Lancet 2019;393:1958–1972.

2 Ho FK, Gray SR, Welsh P, et al: Associations of fat and carbohydrate intake with cardiovascular disease and mortality: prospective cohort study of UK Biobank participants. BMJ 2020;368:m688.

3 Seidelmann SB, Claggett B, Cheng S, et al: Dietary carbohydrate intake and mortality: a prospective cohort study and meta-analysis. Lancet Online 2018;3:e419–e428. www.thelancet.com/publichealth.

4 Astrup A, Magkos F, Bier DM, et al: Saturated fats and health: a reassessment of evidence and proposal for food-based recommendations. J Am Coll Cardiol 2020;76. https://www.onlinejacc.org/content/accj/76/7/844.full.pdf.

5 Mozaffarian D, Hao T, Rimm EB, et al: Changes in diet and lifestyle and long-term weight gain in women and men. N Engl J Med 2011;364:2392–2404.

6 Tan H-E, Sisti AC, Jin H, et al: The gut-brain axis mediates sugar preference. Nature 2020;580:511–516.

7 Owen OE, Morgan AP, Kemp HG, et al: Brain metabolism during fasting. J Clin Invest 1967;46: 1589–1595.

8 Guthrie RA, Guthrie DW, Murthy DYN, et al: Standardization of the oral glucose tolerance test and the criteria for diagnosis of chemical diabetes in children. Metabolism 1973;22:275–282.

9 Knopf CF, Cresto JC, Dujovne IL, et al: Oral glucose tolerance test in 100 normal children. Acta Diabetol Lat 1977;14:95–103.

10 Sunehag AL, Toffolo G, Treuth MS, et al: Effects of dietary macronutrient content on glucose metabolism in children. J Clin Endocrinol Metab 2002;87:5168–5178.

11 Sunehag AL, Toffolo G, Campioni M, et al: Effects of dietary macronutrient intake on insulin sensitivity and secretion and glucose and lipid metabolism in healthy, obese adolescents. J Clin Endocrinol Metab 2005;90:4496–4502.

12 Sunehag AL, Toffolo G, Campioni M, et al: Short-term high dietary fructose intake had no effects on insulin sensitivity and secretion or glucose and lipid metabolism in healthy, obese adolescents. J Pediatr Endocr Metab 2008;21:225–235.

13 Treuth MS, Sunehag AL, Trautwein LM, et al: Metabolic adaptation to high-fat and high-carbohydrate diets in children and adolescents. Am J Clin Nutr 2003;77:479–489.

14 Sunehag AL, Dalla Man C, Toffolo G, et al: β-Cell function and insulin sensitivity in adolescents from an OGTT. Obesity 2008;17:233–239.

15 Stanhope KL, Schwarz JM, Keim NL, et al: Consuming fructose-sweetened, not glucose-sweetened, beverages increases visceral adiposity and lipids and decreases insulin sensitivity in overweight/obese humans. J Clin Invest 2009;119: 1322–1334.

16 Stanhope KL, Medici V, Bremer AA, et al: A dose-response study of consuming high-fructose corn syrup-sweetened beverages on lipid-lipoprotein risk factors for cardiovascular disease in young adults. Am J Clin Nutr 2015;101:1144–1154.

17 Softic S, Stanhope KL, Boucher J, et al: Fructose and hepatic insulin resistance. Crit Rev Clin Lab Sci 2020;14:1–15.

18 Trepanowski JF, Ioannidis JPA: Perspective: limiting dependence on nonrandomized studies and improving randomized trials in human nutrition research: why and how. Adv Nutr 2018;9:367–377.

19 Archer E, Lavie CJ, Hill JO: The failure to measure dietary intake engendered a fictional discourse on diet-disease relations. Front Nutr 2018; 5:105.

20 Archer E, Marlow ML, Lavie CJ: Controversy and debate: memory-based methods paper 2: the fatal flaws of food frequency questionnaires and other memory-based dietary assessment methods. J Clin Epidemiol 2018;104:113–124.

21 Zhong VW, Van Horn L, Greenland P, et al: Associations of processed meat, unprocessed red meat, poultry, or fish intake with incident cardiovascular disease and all-cause mortality. JAMA Intern Med 2020;180:503–512.

22 SACN (Scientific Advisory Committee on Nutrition): Carbohydrates and Health. London, The Stationery Office, 2015.

23 Khan TA, Mobusha T, Agarwal A, et al: Relation of total sugars, sucrose, fructose, and added sugars with the risk of cardiovascular disease: a systematic review and dose-response meta-analysis of prospective cohort studies. Mayo Clin Proc 2019;94:2399–2414.

24 Tsilas CS, de Souza RJ, Blanco Mejia S, et al: Relation of total sugars, fructose and sucrose with incident type 2 diabetes: a systematic review and meta-analysis of prospective cohort studies. CMAJ 2017;189:E711–E720.

25 Jayalath VH, de Souza RJ, Ha V, et al: Sugar-sweetened beverage consumption and incident hypertension: a systematic review and meta-analysis of prospective cohorts. Am J Clin Nutr 2015; 102:914–921.

Published online: November 6, 2020
Black MM, Singhal A, Hillman CH (eds): Building Future Health and Well-Being of Thriving Toddlers and Young Children. Nestlé Nutr Inst Workshop Ser. Basel, Karger, 2020, vol 95, pp 112–115 (DOI: 10.1159/000511526)

Summary on Advancing from Infancy to Toddlerhood through Food

The second session of the workshop, "Advancing from Infancy to Toddlerhood through Food," addresses both the nutritional requirements and the feeding behavior of toddlers. Habits established during toddlerhood that promote healthy dietary choices and self-regulation around eating contribute to healthy growth in toddlerhood, as well as throughout childhood and adolescence. The speakers in this session address both how children learn to eat and what nutrients they are consuming.

The first chapter of this session by Lorrene Ritchie, Danielle L. Lee, Elyse Homel Vitale, and Lauren E. Au is entitled, "Transition from Breastfeeding and Complementary Feeding to *Toddler Nutrition* in Child Care Settings." Ritchie and colleagues developed a procedure to establish nutrition standards to guide feeding young children in licensed child care settings. They begin by noting that 1 in 5 US children are overweight or obese before entering kindergarten, and over one-third of all young children spend time in organized, licensed child care, making child care an optimal setting to promote healthy eating. They also emphasize that nutrition standards are needed to address both what and how to feed young children, including nutrition practices that address the transition from infants to toddlers, that are important for health, and that can be feasibly implemented in child care settings. In the USA, licensed facilities vary from small family child care homes with a single provider and a few children to large centers with a director, multiple teachers, and several hundred children. The goal of Ritchie et al. is to establish a process to develop nutrition standards that are both evidence based and feasible for implementation in all child care settings, including child care homes. Nutrition experts and child care practice-based stakeholders reviewed and modified existing nutrition guidelines and used a Delphi procedure to develop standards. The standards were reviewed by an independent group of child care community advisors for ease of implementation. In the final step, the nutrition standards were pilot tested in 30 licensed family child care providers over 3 months to assess adherence and implementation challenges. The final nutrition standards include not only what foods and beverages to serve but also how to feed infants and toddlers. The next step is to test the standards in a cluster-randomized controlled trial to assess both the feasibility for providers and the impact on child nutrition and weight.

The second chapter by Steven A. Abrams addresses the nutritional needs of toddlers: "Selected Micronutrient Needs of Children 1–3 Years of Age." Abrams reviews the evidence for the key micronutrients needed for growth, neurodevelopment, and immune functioning (iron and zinc) and for bone health (calcium, vitamin D, and magnesium). Some of the methods used to determine toddlers' micronutrient needs are particularly challenging for toddlers because they require stable isotopes, the route of administration is oral or intravenous, and absorption is based on isotopes in the urine.

In industrialized countries, for most toddlers iron intake matches published requirements. In contrast, in several parts of the world, iron deficiency and anemia are common among toddlers. Diets of toddlers are often very low in meat, and fortification of grains is widely done both for iron and zinc. Generally, zinc intakes are above recommendations for most toddlers, particularly in industrialized settings. The calcium requirement is easily achieved for most toddlers with a diet that includes dairy products or fortified-plant-based or other beverages. Vitamin D deficiency is generally low in this age group, but it does exist, and can result in rickets, especially when combined with low calcium intake. Magnesium-deficient intake is relatively uncommon with mixed diets and difficult for clinicians to assess. Future work is needed to determine dietary requirements for vitamins and minerals in small children. This effort needs to be global in scope and account for regional or cultural differences in dietary patterns.

The third chapter by Catherine A. Forestell provides an overview of taste development, perception, and food preferences in young children in a chapter entitled, "You Are What Your Parents Eat: Parental Influences on Early Flavor Preference Development." Forestell reminds us that children consume fewer fruits and vegetables than recommended, and their diets are high in saturated fat, sugar, and salt. Children are predisposed to prefer sweet-tasting foods and beverages, and to avoid bitter-tasting foods such as dark-green vegetables, which reveals the adaptive role of taste from an evolutionary perspective. However, flavor experiences begin prenatally through the olfactory and gustatory systems, and they occur early in life through breastfeeding. Parents continue to influence their children's taste preferences through continued and repeated exposure. Children's likelihood of accepting healthy foods is enhanced by repeated exposure to the flavors of healthy foods and by role modeling from their parents eating healthy foods. Although infants are relatively accepting of new foods soon after weaning, during toddlerhood, many become neophobic or hesitant to accept new foods. Parenting practices that include providing healthy food and ensuring that the setting is supportive and responsive to the child's needs can promote healthy eating. Children's taste preferences are also influenced by environmental conditions, such as food insecurity, limiting the quality and quantity of food available. Forestell describes the Special Supplemental Nutrition Program for Women, Infants, and Children (WIC), a US program that provides food, nutritional counseling, and screening for children under 5 years of age in low-income households.

Susan L. Johnson and Kameron J. Moding present the fourth chapter: "Introducing Hard-to-Like Foods to Infants and Toddlers: Mothers' Perspectives and Children's Experiences about Learning to Accept Novel Foods." Findings from this chapter suggest a "sweet spot" for food introduction and acceptance during the early complementary feeding period (6–12 months of age), with increasing variability in acceptance and negative child behavior occurring during toddlerhood. Strategies to increase children's exposure to novel foods are based on Zajonc's mere exposure theory. Repeated exposure increases children's willingness to try a target food, which then leads to increases in consumption. Another strategy to overcome food refusal is to mix flavors of liked foods with flavors of less-liked or disliked foods based on the principle of associative conditioning. Developing the ability to engage in a novel experience may enhance the development of self-regulation during eating. Responsive parenting and feeding help to promote the development of emotional, social, and cognitive development, and also help young children to learn self-regulation of eating. Johnson and Moding describe the Good Tastes Study, where they recorded mother-child interactions and child responses to a hard-to-like bitter green vegetable (kale). They found that children's refusal increased as they transitioned to toddlerhood. However, the more difficult the feeding, the less mothers persisted in offering the disliked food. Thus, a cycle emerged with children refusing a novel food and mothers limiting their exposure, resulting in persistence of food refusal and lack of self-regulation skills. Promoting self-feeding skills may be an effective strategy to help children increase their willingness to try new foods and promote self-regulation.

The final and fifth chapter of the session by Dennis M. Bier examines associations between sugar intake and health: "Dietary Sugars: Not as Sour as They Are Made Out to Be?" Bier focuses on dietary sugar and the strong feelings and advice that have emerged, linking dietary sugars to obesity and other adverse health conditions, including cardiovascular diseases. He reviews evolutionary evidence that the human body makes necessary sugars, that glucose is essential during fetal development, that the brain prefers glucose for activities, and that infants are born with sweet taste receptors. Although dietary sugar should not be consumed to the point that it contributes to excess energy or displaces the intake of essential nutrients, healthy lean children adjust their internal metabolic mechanisms to accommodate for changes in dietary macronutrient composition. However, children with obesity are less able to adjust their insulin sensitivity in response to a high dietary sugar.

In 2015, the UK Scientific Advisory Committee on Nutrition (UKSACN) published a comprehensive report on carbohydrates and health, which found that dietary sugars were not associated with adverse health conditions, including coronary events, blood pressure, total or LDL cholesterol, fasting triglycerides, fasting glucose or insulin, or the risk of type 2 diabetes mellitus. Although research has shown that most individuals, particularly children who are not obese, can metabolize dietary sugars, warnings against the intake of dietary sugar continue. Bier concluded that sugars in the diet are not as "sour" as they are commonly made out to be.

Maureen M. Black

Published online: November 6, 2020

Black MM, Singhal A, Hillman CH (eds): Building Future Health and Well-Being of Thriving Toddlers and Young Children. Nestlé Nutr Inst Workshop Ser. Basel, Karger, 2020, vol 95, pp 116–126 (DOI: 10.1159/000511508)

A Review of the Effects of Physical Activity on Cognition and Brain Health across Children and Adolescence

Charles H. Hillman[a, b] Katherine M. McDonald[a]
Nicole E. Logan[a]

[a]Department of Psychology, Northeastern University, Boston, MA, USA; [b]Department of Physical Therapy, Movement, and Rehabilitation Sciences, Northeastern University, Boston, MA, USA

Abstract

Physical activity (PA) can improve physical, mental, cognitive, and brain health throughout the lifespan. During preadolescent childhood, the benefits of PA for cognitive health have been widely studied, with evidence indicating enhanced executive control, improved academic performance, and adaptation in underlying brain structure and function. Across school age children, the predominant literature has focused on preadolescent children, with a comparatively smaller body of evidence in adolescent children. Yet, preliminary findings suggest improvements in verbal, numeric, and reasoning abilities as well as academic achievements. Further, benefits of PA are also rarely examined in preschool children. Consequently, lack of standardization across studies has led to various approaches in the measurement of PA and fitness. However, since implementing tools that objectively quantify active play, PA has been related to better executive function, language acquisition, and academic achievement. Despite evidence that PA promotes cognitive and brain health during development, a growing number of schools have minimized PA opportunities across the school day. The minimization of PA along with several other factors, including lack of active commuting to school, nutrition transition, and availability of electronic devices, for example, has reduced children's physical and mental health. Accordingly, today's children have become increasingly inactive, which affects public health and contributes to educational concerns. By dedicating time to active play, sports, physical education, and other forms of PA, children are best positioned to thrive in both the physical and cognitive domains.

Introduction

Despite recommendations and widespread health campaigns from the World Health Organization [1] and the 2018 Physical Activity Guidelines for Americans [2] aimed at improving health and wellness among youth, most children are not adequately physically active to derive the full health benefits. In fact, less than 24% of children aged 6–17 years engage in the recommended 60+ min of daily moderate-to-vigorous physical activity (MVPA) [3]. Physical activity (PA) behaviors during childhood track into adolescence and adulthood [4], which is concerning since physical inactivity has been linked to earlier mortality and greater morbidity associated with multiple chronic diseases [2]. Largely absent from these public health concerns is the effect of physical inactivity on cognitive and brain health. Further, many school districts have obviated PA from the school day due to budgetary constraints and an increased emphasis placed on standardized test performance. Although it may seem counterintuitive that spending less time in the classroom and more time engaged in PA might serve to improve cognition and learning [5], there is a growing literature detailing the beneficial effects of PA on brain health, cognition, and academic performance [6].

The current literature on the benefits of PA for brain and cognition differ across youth. Specifically, the majority of evidence exists among preadolescent children (6–13 years) [6], with comparatively less research in preschool children [7] and adolescents [8]. Although the extant findings overwhelmingly indicate benefits of PA on brain structure and function as well as cognition and academic performance, outstanding research questions remain. Accordingly, this article summarizes the current literature on the benefits of PA for brain health and cognition in youth, and highlights future areas of research needed to advance the state of the science.

Preschool Children

Early childhood is a critical period of motor, mental, and cognitive health development [2]. PA has been shown to act on and improve different health outcomes in children, but to date, physical health outcomes have been researched more commonly than mental and cognitive health outcomes in children younger than 6 years [7]. Considering the importance of this period of rapid growth, investigating the potential effects of PA on cognition and brain health in this population is imperative.

Brain development begins in the first trimester of pregnancy, accelerates postnatally through the second year, and continues throughout the lifespan [9]. Cognitive health in children younger than 2 years is largely tethered to the achievement of behavioral milestones such as attending to faces, reacting to sounds in the environment, smiling, speaking, or playing with toys at appropriate time points of development [10]. PA for children under 2 years can be strengthening neck muscles to hold their head up, rolling over, stretching their legs and arms, and learning to sit up, crawl, and walk [10]. Although the quantifiable connection between cognitive health and PA in children under 2 years of age remains unknown, it is generally thought that novel experiences that promote motor skills, movement, and exploration enhance neuroplasticity and further cognitive growth [9].

In children between 3 and 5 years, the most prevalent form of PA is active play. Given that active play is naturally unstructured, standardization of PA measures in this age group is difficult to obtain [11]. In recent years, there has been a shift away from subjective reporting to using pedometers and accelerometers that capture objective daily PA (i.e., step counts) [11]. Using accelerometers, it has been suggested that young children who spend more time in MVPA during play showed improvements in self-regulation – an encompassing term used to describe integrated executive functioning capabilities such as inhibitory control, working memory, and cognitive flexibility [12]. More broadly, systematic reviews have concluded that young children who participate in greater amounts of PA have demonstrated improvements in executive function, language acquisition, and academic achievement [7].

Fitness is also challenging to measure in this demographic. The gold standard laboratory measure for fitness is a graded exercise ($\text{VO}_{2\,\text{max}}$) test, during which a participant typically runs/walks on a treadmill or cycles on an ergometer until volitional exhaustion. $\text{VO}_{2\,\text{max}}$ testing has been successfully completed in children as young as 4 years, but it is subject to physical limitations of the individual – children shorter than 125 cm may require a pediatric treadmill or cycle ergometer [13]. Additionally, there is debate whether children achieve a true $\text{VO}_{2\,\text{max}}$, which occurs during a plateau of oxygen uptake [13]. Although $\text{VO}_{2\,\text{max}}$ has been positively related to daily activity variables captured via accelerometry in children younger than 6 years, the relationship was only found in boys, contradicting previous studies in older children and adolescents [14].

The lack of standardized measures has yielded diverse approaches to quantifying fitness in young children. For example, isolated physical fitness measures such as muscular strength, running speed, balance, flexibility, and coordination are inconsistently measured and reported in this population [15]. Field-based fitness tests such as a shuttle run to measure aerobic fitness, obstacle courses to measure motor skills, and balance beams to measure dynamic balance have been associated with better attention and spatial working memory [16].

Additional efforts have been made to connect other easily measurable health indicators, such as weight status, to cognition in children. While the effects of obesity on brain health in children younger than 6 years are inconclusive, higher body fat percentage is associated with poorer executive control and academic achievement in youth slightly older than preschool children (6–8 years) [17].

Overall, current knowledge regarding the benefits of PA for cognition and brain health in preschool children suffers from variability of measurement, and given that the field is currently emerging, there are important considerations moving forward. Recent interest in this demographic has suggested that maintaining a healthy lifestyle, including engaging in regular PA and maintaining a healthy body mass, should be established early in childhood to capitalize on benefits for cognition and brain health across the lifespan.

School Age Children

Preadolescent Children

As PA continues to decrease throughout the lifespan, critical populations of interest include preadolescent and adolescent demographics. The physical inactivity epidemic is widespread, affecting not only US children. Comparably, European preadolescent children spend only 16 min/day (5%) in MVPA but 209 min/day (64%) engaged in sedentary activities [18]. Given that PA behaviors during preadolescent childhood track into adolescence and adulthood [4], early intervention is necessary to positively promote greater participation in PA across the lifespan, subsequently leading to the promotion of healthier lifestyles.

The benefits of PA intervention in preadolescent children are extensive, encompassing many aspects of physical, mental, cognitive, and brain health. For example, PA interventions are efficacious for enhancing mental health and wellness [19], increasing executive control [20–23], and improving academic performance [21, 23] in preadolescent children. In recent years, a move towards understanding the cognitive and underlying brain structure and function mechanistic relationship in response to PA interventions has emerged. PA dose-response relationships in preadolescent children have indicated that higher attendance in an afterschool PA program is associated with larger changes in neural indices of attention and processing speed, as measured by event-related brain potentials, and improved performance during tasks of executive control and academic performance (Fig. 1a, b) [21]. Specifically, children in the FITKids and FITKids2 clinical trials delivered a 2-h PA intervention during 5 school days per week for

9 months (150 days), based on the Child and Adolescent Trial for Cardiovascular Health (CATCH) curriculum, which provided MVPA in an after-school noncompetitive environment. Children who were randomized to the PA intervention were compared before and after the test to children who were randomly allocated to the wait list control group. This control group was asked to maintain their regular after-school routine and were not contacted again until 9 months after testing.

Overall, when examining the preadolescent brain responses to PA, children demonstrated enhanced cognitive performance and brain function during tasks requiring greater amounts of executive control (i.e., tasks that modulated inhibition, working memory, and cognitive flexibility demands) at the 9-month post-test, relative to before the test, and this effect was absent for children assigned to the control group [20–22]. Moreover, the observed behavioral benefits coincided with interesting brain (i.e., event-related brain potentials) outcomes, such that children in the PA intervention exhibited a larger P3 amplitude (Fig. 1a), stability of the error-related negativity potential (Fig. 1c), and a larger initial contingent negative variation amplitude (Fig. 1d) compared to children in the control group 9 months after the test. Such findings suggest that the PA intervention was beneficial to brain functions underlying the allocation of attentional resources, conflict monitoring, and cognitive preparation processes during tasks that require executive functions, respectively. Lastly, increased aerobic fitness, which is associated with increased levels of PA, was found to correlate with tasks of inhibitory control and academic achievement [23].

Furthermore, recent evidence has suggested that PA is associated with increased white matter microstructure in the genu (the anterior bulbar end of the corpus callosum) [24]. Specifically, the 9-month FITKids trial demonstrated that children in the PA intervention showed increases in fractional anisotropy (the total magnitude of directional movement along axonal fibers) and decreas-

Fig. 1. Data from the FITKids and FITKids2 trials illustrating cognitive and brain changes stemming from a 9-month PA intervention compared to a wait list control group in preadolescent children. **a** Topographic scalp plots demonstrating mean change in P3 amplitude (μV) during modified flanker and switch tasks for each group [21]. **b** Response accuracy (%) for the modified flanker task, and the homogeneous and heterogeneous conditions of the switch task for each group and time point [21]. **c** Topographic scalp plots depicting the mean change in error-related negativity amplitude (μV) during the modified flanker task for each group [20]. **d** Topographic scalp plots demonstrating an initial contingent negative variation amplitude for each group and time point [22]. **e** The ratio of fractional anisotropy (FA) and radial diffusivity (RD) for the genu of the corpus callosum (mm^2/s) for each group and time point [24]. **f** Mean percent change in the blood oxygen level-dependent signal for the right anterior prefrontal cortex (PFC) and incongruent flanker task response accuracy (%) for each group and time point [25].

es in radial diffusivity (a sensitive measure for axonal or myelin damage, defined as the magnitude of diffusion perpendicular to the tract) in the genu after the test compared to before the test – an observation which was not seen in the control group (Fig. 1e). Importantly, the genu of the corpus callosum is an area associated with the integration of cognitive, motor, and sensory information be-

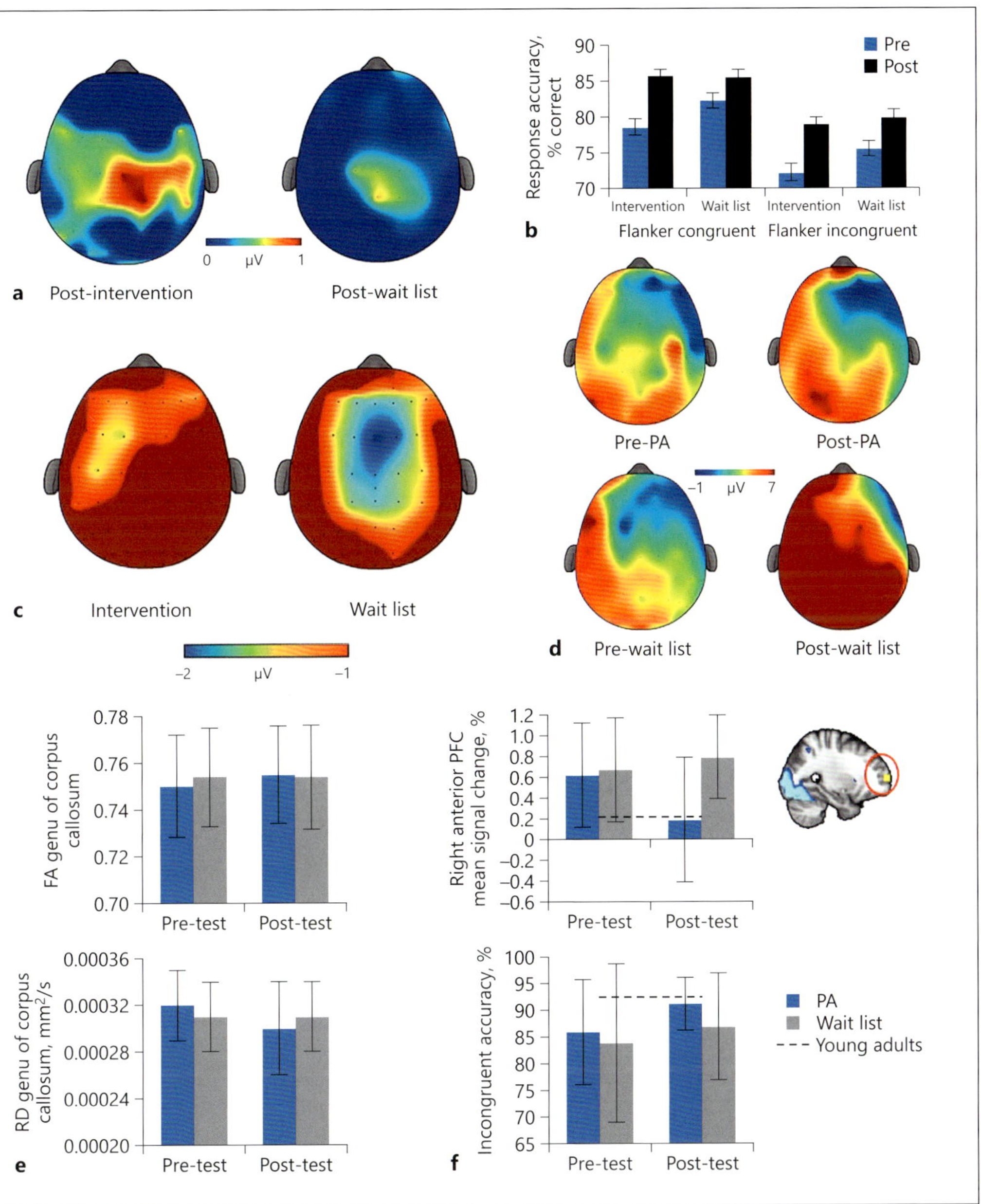

tween the left and right hemispheres of the brain. Notably, the FITKids trial also revealed that children in the PA intervention showed decreased brain activation, as measured via functional MRI, in the right anterior prefrontal cortex, coupled with within-group performance improvements in an inhibitory control task (Fig. 1f) [25]. Collectively, functional MRI data suggest that PA and fitness are important lifestyle factors for cognitive and brain health in preadolescent children. The FITKids clinical trials further indicate that daily PA serves to increase aerobic fitness alongside improvements in academic performance, executive function, and underlying brain structure and function. Meanwhile, such findings were not demonstrated in a control group of children following 9 months of typical development.

Adolescent Children

In addition to research focused on child and preadolescent populations, the relationship between adolescent cognitive performance and brain outcomes in response to PA has recently attracted investigative focus; however, the field is relatively unexplored compared to the extant literature with preadolescent children. Specifically, cross-sectional studies have explored this relationship in adolescents, and data suggest that children who participated in PA during extracurricular leisure time had better cognitive performance on measures of verbal, numeric, and reasoning ability [26]. Further, apart from extracurricular activities, better cognitive performance across similar measures was observed in adolescent females who reported actively commuting to school (e.g., walking or biking) compared to nonactive adolescent female commuters (e.g., car, bus, or subway) [27]. These cross-sectional studies, which delve into cognitive responses to healthy PA behaviors, have initiated a framework for further investigation, and collectively provide evidence of a positive relationship between PA and cognitive function [8]. Evidently, there is a need for chronic PA interventions in adolescents, across the entire school day, to appropriately assess the effects of PA on brain and cognition.

Lastly, the effects of PA interventions on academic achievement have also been explored. Specifically, an in-school vigorous PA intervention over the course of 1 semester was associated with higher grades in academic achievement at the completion of the semester [28]. Notably, the increased grades were not observed in children who participated in moderate PA interventions, suggesting that this effect was only related to the PA of vigorous intensity [28]. Additionally, an acute in-school PA intervention in adolescents demonstrated increased performance in mathematical tasks, indicating that benefits may be observed immediately following the cessation of an exercise bout, as well as following prolonged exposure to PA behaviors. [29]. Collectively, these data suggest enhanced academic performance in response to PA interventions in both preadolescent and adolescent children. As school districts continue to move away from PA opportunities during the school day due to budgetary constraints and an increased emphasis on standardized test performance, these trends on the beneficial effects of PA for brain health, cognition, and academic performance of school-age children are important to consider [6].

Future Directions

There are certainly a number of important future directions that are necessary to advance the field of childhood PA, brain health, and cognition. Compared to preschool-age children (<6 years), efforts must be directed toward improving the precision of data collection both in terms of exposure variables, such as the measurement of PA behaviors, and in terms of the measurement of cognitive outcomes. That is, the field has yet to develop consensus on the best means for measuring PA in younger children. Further, there are a number of tests available to assess cognition during this period of development, yet much of the existing PA literature has lacked a theoretically guided approach, with little understanding of development and maturation. For example, given that preschool-age children are undergoing rapid maturation, research in this area should consider timing PA interventions with critical periods of development, a window during which the brain is most responsive (i.e., open to structuring and restructuring) to environmental exposures. Similar consideration for critical periods has been used with other behavioral interventions, such as for optimizing language acquisition [30]. It is plausible that brain and cognition may be especially amenable to PA intervention during specific critical periods affording greater opportunity to provide health benefits to preschool-age children.

Compared to school-age children (6–18 years), the study of PA on brain and cognition has developed more rapidly, with more sophisticated study intervention designs and measurement approaches to assess brain and cognition. However, considerably more research is necessary to unpack the underlying neural mechanisms that underpin cognitive enhancements. For example, we are just beginning to understand changes in neural networks, rather than single regions or areas of the brain, that are influenced by PA behavior. Future research will need to combine these neural network approaches to understanding modifications in the whole brain with randomized controlled trials that offer the sophistication and proper controls to afford causal evidence. The further ability to link PA-induced changes in neural networks that underlie academic performance is an additional future direction that is ripe for study.

A final future direction that warrants further consideration is individual differences in PA effects on brain and cognition. That is, individual differences in response to PA intervention are common, but with respect to brain and cognition, little is known regarding what underlies differential responses. Previous findings in the literature indicate differential responses as a function of sex, genetic makeup, body composition, and disability/disease status, to name only a few. A systematic approach to understanding individual differences and their influence on the effects of PA on brain and cognition is imperative toward designing effective interventions aimed at improving public health.

Conclusion

The importance of PA on early cognitive and brain health and development in children is evident. Data suggest a beneficial relationship between the time preschool children spent in MVPA through active play (assessed by means of accelerometry) and greater improvements in measures of self-regulation. Additionally, the positive effects of PA on cognitive and brain health in older children are vast. PA interventions in preadolescent children have demonstrated greater improvements in neural indices of attention, conflict monitoring, motor preparation, and processing speed, as well as improved performance during tasks of executive control and academic performance. Neuroimaging data also indicate greater improvements in executive control tasks coupled with decreased activation in the right anterior prefrontal cortex.

Further, cross-sectional adolescent research has demonstrated the importance of considering the effects of PA on fitness and cognitive and brain outcomes. Importantly, adolescents who participate in greater amounts of PA demonstrate greater performance on measures of verbal, numeric, and reasoning ability. Meanwhile, in-school intervention data suggest vigorous PA over the course of just 1 semester is associated with better performance in academic achievement tasks. Collectively, both structured and unstructured PA throughout development is essential to promote cognitive and brain health in children.

PA is important to consider when evaluating and promoting the health and development of all children. Recently, many school districts have focused their curriculum toward spending more time in the classroom and less time engaged in PA. However, evidence suggests this may in fact be counterintuitive to the improvement in classroom-based learning, as PA positively promotes cognitive and brain health and academic performance. Consequently, restructuring classroom time to include regular bouts of PA throughout the school day is recommended. PA trends have also demonstrated that healthy behaviors during childhood track into adulthood. Thus, implementing healthy behaviors early during development and throughout the school curriculum is likely to positively influence the adherence of PA across the lifespan. Habitual commitment to PA is therefore important for the public health of children as they develop into adulthood, as well as when considering the health behaviors of subsequent generations.

Conflict of Interest Statement

The authors declare no conflict of interest.

Funding Sources

The author did not receive funding for the development of this article.

References

1 World Health Organization: Physical Activity and Young People. Geneva, WHO, 2011.

2 Physical Activity Guidelines Advisory Committee: 2018 Physical Activity Guidelines Advisory Committee Scientific Report. Washington, US Department of Health and Human Services, 2018.

3 National Physical Activity Plan Alliance: The 2018 United States Report Card on Physical Activity for Children and Youth. Washington, National Physical Activity Plan Alliance, 2018.

4 Kjønniksen L, Torsheim T, Wold B: Tracking of leisure-time physical activity during adolescence and young adulthood: a 10-year longitudinal study. Int J Behav Nutr Phys Act 2008;5:69.

5 Sallis JF: We do not have to sacrifice children's health to achieve academic goals. J Pediatr 2010; 156:696–697.

6 Donnelly JE, Hillman CH, Castelli D, et al: Physical activity, fitness, cognitive function, and academic achievement in children: a systematic review. Med Sci Sports Exerc 2016;48:1197–1222.

7 Pate RR, Hillman CH, Janz KF, et al: Physical activity and health in children younger than 6 years: a systematic review. Med Sci Sports Exerc 2019;51:1282–1291.

8 Esteban-Cornejo I, Tejero-Gonzalez CM, Sallis JF, Veiga OL: Physical activity and cognition in adolescents: a systematic review. J Sci Med Sport 2015;18:534–539.

9 Mundkur N: Neuroplasticity in children. Indian J Pediatr 2005;72:855–857.

10 Growth and Development; in Trubo R, Shelov SP, Hannemann RE, et al. (eds): Caring for Your Baby and Young Child: Birth to Age Five, ed 4. New York, Bantam, 2004, pp 143–364.

11 Knowles G, Pallan M, Thomas GN, et al: Physical activity and blood pressure in primary school children: a longitudinal study. Hypertension 2013;61:70–75.

12 Becker DR, Mcclelland MM, Loprinzi PD, Trost S: Physical activity, self-regulation, and early academic achievement in preschool children. Early Educ Dev 2014;25:56–70.

13 Takken T, Bongers BC, van Brussel M, et al: Cardiopulmonary exercise testing in pediatrics. Ann Am Thorac Soc 2017;14(suppl 1):123–128.

14 Dencker M, Bugge A, Hermansen B, Andersen LB: Objectively measured daily physical activity related to aerobic fitness in young children. J Sports Sci 2010;28:139–145.

15 Wang H, Wu D, Zhang Y, et al: The association of physical growth and behavior change with preschooler's physical fitness: from 10-years of monitoring data. J Exerc Sci Fit 2019;17:113–118.

16 Niederer I, Kriemler S, Gut J, et al: Relationship of aerobic fitness and motor skills with memory and attention in preschoolers (Ballabeina): a cross-sectional and longitudinal study. BMC Pediatr 2011;11:34.

17 Kamijo K, Khan NA, Pontifex MB, et al: The relation of adiposity to cognitive control and scholastic achievement in preadolescent children. Obesity (Silver Spring) 2012;20:2406–2411.

18 van Stralen MM, Yıldırım M, Wulp A, et al: Measured sedentary time and physical activity during the school day of European 10- to 12-year-old children: the ENERGY project. J Sci Med Sport 2014;17:201–206.
19 Rodriguez-Ayllon M, Cadenas-Sánchez C, Estévez-López F, et al: Role of physical activity and sedentary behavior in the mental health of preschoolers, children and adolescents: a systematic review and meta-analysis. Sports Med 2019;49: 1383–1410.
20 Drollette ES, Pontifex MB, Raine LB, et al: Effects of the FITKids physical activity randomized controlled trial on conflict monitoring in youth. Psychophysiology 2018;55:10.1111/psyp.13017.
21 Hillman CH, Pontifex MB, Castelli DM, et al: Effects of the FITKids randomized controlled trial on executive control and brain function. Pediatrics 2014;134:e1063–e1071.
22 Kamijo K, Pontifex MB, O'Leary KC, et al: The effects of an afterschool physical activity program on working memory in preadolescent children. Dev Sci 2011;14:1046–1058.
23 Pindus DM, Drollette ES, Scudder MR, et al: Moderate-to-vigorous physical activity, indices of cognitive control, and academic achievement in preadolescents. J Pediatr 2016;173:136–142.
24 Chaddock-Heyman L, Erickson KI, Kienzler C, et al: Physical activity increases white matter microstructure in children. Front Neurosci 2018;12: 950.
25 Chaddock-Heyman L, Erickson KI, Voss MW, et al: The effects of physical activity on functional MRI activation associated with cognitive control in children: a randomized controlled intervention. Front Hum Neurosci 2013;7:72.
26 Ruiz JR, Ortega FB, Castillo R, et al: Physical activity, fitness, weight status, and cognitive performance in adolescents. J Pediatr 2010;157:917–922.e1–5.
27 Martínez-Gómez D, Ruiz JR, Gómez-Martínez S, et al; AVENA Study Group: Active commuting to school and cognitive performance in adolescents: the AVENA study. Arch Pediatr Adolesc Med 2011;165:300–305.
28 Coe DP, Pivarnik JM, Womack CJ, et al: Effect of physical education and activity levels on academic achievement in children. Med Sci Sports Exerc 2006;38:1515–1519.
29 Travlos AK: High intensity physical education classes and cognitive performance in eighth-grade students: an applied study. Int J Sport Exerc Psychol 2010;8:302–311.
30 Werker JF, Hensch TK: Critical periods in speech perception: new directions. J Annu Rev Psychol 2015;66:173–196.

Published online: November 9, 2020

Black MM, Singhal A, Hillman CH (eds): Building Future Health and Well-Being of Thriving Toddlers and Young Children. Nestlé Nutr Inst Workshop Ser. Basel, Karger, 2020, vol 95, pp 127–135 (DOI: 10.1159/000511513)

Nutrition Effects on Childhood Executive Control

Nathaniel Willis[a] Naiman A. Khan[a–c]

[a]Division of Nutritional Sciences, University of Illinois at Urbana-Champaign, Urbana, IL, USA; [b]Department of Kinesiology and Community Health, University of Illinois at Urbana-Champaign, Urbana, IL, USA; [c]Neuroscience Program, University of Illinois at Urbana-Champaign, Urbana, IL, USA

Abstract

Greater abilities for executive control in childhood have long-term benefits for academic and vocational success. Therefore, lifestyle approaches with the potential to support executive control in childhood stand to have long-term implications not only for physical but also for cognitive health. Nutrition plays a fundamental role in brain structure and function. While a considerable amount of literature demonstrates the detrimental effects of deficiencies in essential nutrients, comparatively little is known is about the role of overall diet quality in promoting executive control among children without diagnosed nutrient deficiencies. Emerging evidence provides preliminary support for the importance of key nutrients (e.g., water, dietary fiber, carotenoids, and choline) that contribute to diet quality. This article represents a brief narrative review that aims to highlight the importance of habitual diet quality for executive control in childhood. Additional research is needed to continue developing the evidence base for diet patterns and nutrients that preferentially support executive control during childhood. This is an important goal given that nutritional recommendations for children's cognitive function are absent from the US dietary guidelines, making the endeavor to develop the evidence base for diet patterns and nutrients that preferentially support executive control during childhood all the more important.

Introduction

Individuals with greater ability for executive control, also known as executive functions (i.e., inhibitory control, working memory, and cognitive flexibility), are more likely to have a higher quality of life across several domains of personal and professional success [1]. Given that childhood is an important period for brain growth and development, lifestyle approaches with the potential to promote executive control could have a lasting impact on children's long-term cognitive health. Specifically, improving diet quality may provide an efficacious target for interventions that aim to positively impact aspects of executive control. Preclinical studies have demonstrated that deficiencies in essential lipids, amino acids, minerals, and vitamins can lead to severe decrements in brain structure and poorer cognitive function [2]. However, while there has been a considerable accumulation of literature demonstrating the detrimental effects of deficiencies in essential nutrients, comparatively little is known is about the role of diet quality in promoting executive control among children without diagnosed nutrient deficiencies. Emerging literature has focused on key nutrients that may play an important role in neural development and physiological health. A comprehensive review of the numerous essential and nonessential nutrients that comprise brain structure and support the myriad of cognitive functions is beyond the scope of any one article. Therefore, this article is focused on a brief narrative review that aims to highlight the importance of specific nutrients (e.g., water, dietary fiber, carotenoids, and choline), known to reflect habitual diet quality, for executive control in childhood.

Lutein

Carotenoids are a diverse class of orange, yellow, and red lipophilic pigments present in many fruits and vegetables, as well as some animal food sources such as eggs. Some carotenoids contribute to vitamin A formation, serving functions in vision, epithelial cell regeneration, and gene expression [3]. Carotenoids also reduce the risk of chronic diseases such as cancers, cardiovascular diseases, and age-related macular degeneration [4]. Lutein and its isomer zeaxanthin are both examples of non-provitamin A carotenoids known as xanthophylls. These xanthophylls and the lutein metabolite *meso*-zeaxanthin comprise the macular pigment, playing important roles as blue-light filters and in countering the exceedingly high oxidative stress in the retina [4]. Relative to other carotenoids, lutein disproportionately accumulates across different regions of the infant brain, including the prefrontal cortex and hippocampus, indicating a particularly important role in the development and function of neural tissue [5]. At molecular level, lutein is uniquely positioned to ameliorate oxidative stress with the presence of terminal hydroxyl groups. The molecule is believed to embed in neural tissue membranes, allowing the terminal polar groups to protect against the oxidation of vulnerable lipids [4].

One of the earliest opportunities to augment lutein status in children is through mother's milk or fortified infant formula. Preclinical work has shown lutein deposition in the brain of breastfed infant macaques to be up to 5 times higher (depending on the location) than in those fed a carotenoid-supplemented formula, demonstrating the importance of lutein for maternal nutrition [6]. Among human infants, a double-blind trial revealed that the human milk group had a sixfold higher geometric mean serum lutein than the unfortified and fortified formula groups, further substantiating the higher bioavailability of lutein in human breast milk [7]. On the other end of the age spectrum, increased macular pigment optical density (MPOD) has long been associated with improved visual performance and has been impactful in delaying the effects of age-related macular degeneration.

The retinal mechanisms are multifaceted but widely believed to be twofold: (1) lutein and zeaxanthin absorb and filter short-wave light protecting the macula from damage and (2) improve neurophysiology by potentially reducing myelin oxidation and allowing for more efficient communication among neurons [4]. Further, MPOD is a strong correlate of brain lutein concentration and provides a noninvasive approach to studying lutein effects on brain and cognitive functions. Lutein and zeaxanthin supplementation studies in adults have consistently demonstrated benefits for MPOD and executive control processes in young as well as older adults [8–10]. Pertinent to the literature in children, MPOD, assessed using a customized heterochromatic flicker photometry approach, can be measured with moderate reliability in preadolescent children as well as adults [11]. Among preadolescent children, MPOD has been positively correlated to subject-specific tests of reading, math, and written language, as well as overall academic achievement [12] and accuracy on a modified flanker task [13], and negatively correlated to task performance (error rate) in a relational memory task [14]. Although intervention trials are lacking in children, the emerging cross-sectional studies in children provide preliminary support for the importance of neural lutein status on executive control, making a compelling case for rigorous experimental approaches in future studies.

Choline

Choline is a nutrient, much like lutein, that exerts a neuroprotective and developmental function through both structural and functional roles. Choline is required for endogenous synthesis of the neurotransmitter acetylcholine and the membrane components phosphatidylcholine and sphingomyelin [15]. Within the myelin sheath, phosphatidylcholine is a primary membrane lipid, and choline-deficient diets have been linked to a reduction in both circulating phosphatidylcholine and neural processing speed [16]. Additionally, declining cholinergic neurotransmission and membrane integrity are both processes that have been implicated in degenerative diseases such as Alzheimer disease [15].

While important for neurological health throughout the life cycle, choline may play a particularly important role in development. Myelination begins during the latter stages of gestation, accelerates through the first 2–3 postnatal years, and continues into early adulthood [16]. A recent double-blind, randomized, controlled study observed that third-trimester maternal choline supplementation (930 mg/day) improved infant's performance on an attention task through the first 15 months of life [17]. This task was previously shown to be predictive of information processing speed and IQ in childhood [17]. Furthermore, there was evidence in the low-intake group indicating that even slight increases in choline intake during pregnancy may have lasting effects on children [17].

Recent work from our laboratory suggests that the beneficial influence of dietary choline on executive control processes is evident even among young adults [18]. Specifically, dietary choline was associated with more efficient neural processing among a sample of overweight and obese adults, as indicated by a lower peak amplitude of the P300 waveform during incongruent trials of a modified Eriksen flanker task. While this is a cross-sectional finding, it is suggestive of the potential role that choline plays in cognitive health throughout life.

Much of the research in dietary or supplement interventions with choline focus on the effects in gestational or geriatric periods – an approach supported by knowledge of the importance of choline in both the structural development of the myelin sheath during pregnancy and the role that abnormal methylation could play in neurodegeneration. However, additional experimental intervention studies are needed to investigate the effects of choline consumption throughout childhood and adolescence as it is unclear whether meeting daily needs for choline in later childhood provides added benefits for cognitive function.

Water

The human body contains 55–75% water, comprising a significant proportion of body composition at the tissue and cellular level. Adequate water intake is crucial to sustaining vital physiological functions, including the transportation of oxygen, nutrients, and waste products. However, evidence from across the globe suggests that the majority of children are chronically dehydrated or insufficiently hydrated. In fact, a recent systematic review showed that on average 60 ± 24% of children failed to meet water intake guidelines of their respective countries [19]. Similarly, recent work from our laboratory has shown that the ad libitum urine concentration of children is quite low. Children in this study exhibited a urine osmolality at baseline that was remarkably similar to their urine osmolality during the water restriction condition (<500 mL of plain water per day) [20]. This is concerning and suggests that children may already be undergoing physiological adaptations to chronic suboptimal hydration.

Water restriction induces hypovolemia which affects peripheral blood flow. In mice, 24-h water deprivation disrupts cerebrovascular regulation and induces cognitive deficits [21]. Further, dehydration increases plasma osmolality, encouraging the osmotic transfer of water out of tissues. Studies have shown that dehydration could potentially reduce brain volume as water is extracted from brain cells into the blood with an inevitable compensatory enlargement of the ventricles [21, 22]. Kempton et al. [22] showed ventricular enlargement proportional to body weight loss following an exercise dehydration protocol in adolescents. Further, while the authors found no significant differences in the performance of a Tower of London task based on hydration status, functional MRI showed increased blood flow to the frontal lobe in the dehydrated state, which is indicative of an increased resource demand to reach the same level of performance.

Understanding the implications of insufficient hydration on cognitive function in children is particularly important since children have a higher surface/mass ratio, which puts them at greater risk of increased loss of body water. Further, children are reliant on caretakers regarding opportunities for drinking water. Findings from our recent 3-condition crossover hydration intervention in children showed that higher water intake was selectively related to improvements in cognitive flexibility and working memory [3]. Specifically, higher working memory cost was observed during the low intake condition (<500 mL/day) when compared to the high intake condition (>2,500 mL/day). These findings were broadly consistent with previous work indicating the benefits of water consumption for cognitive function in school-age children. Overall, such findings suggest adequate hydration may benefit complex cognitive operations. Given that these aspects of cognitive function underlie academic achievement, it is promising that low-cost lifestyle interventions, such as increasing water intake, may benefit effective functioning throughout the school day. However, much of the literature has focused on the detrimental effects of dehydration for cognitive function. Therefore, additional water intervention studies are needed in children with insufficient habitual hydration to better elucidate the health benefits of improved hydration.

Dietary Fibers

Dietary fibers are indigestible carbohydrate polymers, which are neither digested nor absorbed [23]. Increasing dietary fiber has been linked to lowering of a myriad of disease risk factors, including blood pressure and serum cholesterol, while improving glycemia and insulin sensitivity [24] with similar benefits for children as well as adults. Additionally, dietary fibers are subjected to bacterial fermentation [23], impacting the composition of bacterial communities as well as microbial metabolic activities in the gastrointestinal tract. As the gut-microbiota-brain axis incorporates elements of the central, autonomic, and enteric nervous systems, the immune system, and the endocrine system, modulation of the gastrointestinal microbiota by dietary fiber could impact cognitive and brain health via several pathways. Indeed, the microbiome – the term used to refer to the microbial organisms in the gut and their collective genome – has been shown to be cross-sectionally related to human behavior, mental health, body composition, and cognition [25]. The bacteria in the human gut exist in symbiosis, metabolizing indigestible fibers to produce products that can be further absorbed by the host. These endpoints include short- and branched-chain fatty acids, vitamins and minerals, neurotransmitters (serotonin, GABA, and histamine), and many others in smaller concentration [25, 26]. It is also important to note that the microbial communities in the human gut are directly influenced by diet and can be modulated in the short term by dietary interventions [25].

Modulation of gastrointestinal microbiota by indigestible carbohydrates is evident in early life [27]. Preclinical work has shown a positive impact of nondigestible human milk oligosaccharides on hippocampal function and long-term potentiation in rodents [28]. For most mammals, the ingestion of mother's milk is the first case of oral intake of food, and human milk oligosaccharides are important for fueling the newborn microbiome. There is, however, little evidence as to the impact of the human infant's microbiome on cognitive development. This is especially challenging due to the fluctuations in gut microbe communities up until around 2 years of age when an infant generally transitions to solid foods [27].

In prepubertal children, total dietary fiber consumption from a 3-day diet record was shown to be positively associated with attentional inhibition assessed using a modified flanker task [29]. Further, insoluble fiber and pectin intakes (two types of dietary fiber that would be particularly available to gut microbiota) were positively correlated with the task condition placing greater demands on inhibitory control. These findings suggest that fiber intake may be influential in the upregulation of cognitive control in childhood. However, this was a cross-sectional study that did not include assessment of the gastrointestinal microbiome. Therefore, the potential microbiome-dependent mechanisms by which dietary fiber impacts on cognitive function in preadolescent children warrant further examination.

At the latter end of the life cycle, it is thought that the gastrointestinal microbial community decreases and interpersonal variability increases [26]. Intervention studies on fiber supplementation are few and have shown mixed results with some studies reporting positive effects on mood, memory, and executive control in adults while others have shown no effect [30]. Focusing specifically on the microbiome, observational studies in elderly patients have revealed correlations between the relative abundance of gut microbes and cognitive performance such that performance was negatively correlated with Enterobacteriaceae and positively correlated with Lactobacillales. Further, recent findings in patients with Alzheimer disease suggest a microbiome characterized by an overpresence of gram-negative bacteria [26].

The potential mechanisms of interaction are widespread and include modulation of peripheral neural pathways, vagal nerve stimulation, inhibition of the HPA axis, direct effects on blood-brain barrier permeability, absorption of bacterial toxins, and epigenetic mechanisms [25]. Most relevant to diet and cognition: short-chain fatty acids, specifically butyrate, play a direct role in blood-brain barrier permeability, epigenetic modulation of gene transcription in the brain, and the promotion of neurotransmitter and hormone synthesis, as well as the absorption of bacterial toxin, which promotes the production of proinflammatory cytokines resulting in neuroinflammation, apoptosis, and amyloid deposition [25, 26]. These pathways are thought to work in opposition such that a healthy diet may foster a healthier microbial ratio and encourage protective effects via butyrate production – serving to inhibit toxin absorption, reduce systemic and neural inflammation, and delay neurodegeneration.

Gut microbiota is relatively transient given its susceptibility to dietary variations, illness, infections, and pharmacotherapies. We are still at the early stages of understanding exact mechanisms, but the work to elucidate the role of butyrate in ameliorating neurodegeneration is promising [26]. Furthermore, there is compelling evidence supporting the involvement of the gut-brain axis across the life cycle. Dietary modulation of the microbiome using dietary fiber may be involved in influencing the development of the immune system and metabolic pathways in infancy, while also contributing to cognitive function in childhood and protecting against neurodegeneration in later life.

Conclusion

Children are in a period of development to establish habits that can be predictive of future health and are poised to optimize potential for growth. Nutritional intake at this stage is a potent moderator of health. Furthermore, some nutrients discussed here (i.e., carotenoids, choline, water, and dietary fiber) could play a major role in the proper development of neural tissue, the amelioration of cognitive decline, and efficient regulation of cognitive resources. Whereas there is potential of these nutrients to promote executive control, the literature has several limitations. First, a limited number of randomized, controlled trials and a large heterogeneity of cognitive tasks employed present challenges in terms of establishing causality and gaining insights into the specificity of the nutrient effects. Further, the potential mechanisms are largely untested, and future work should strive to elucidate these pathways. Finally, an evidence base needs to be established for specific dietary patterns and nutrients that affect childhood development. This is of special importance as nutritional recommendations for cognitive health of children are absent from the US dietary guidelines.

Conflict of Interest Statement

The authors declare no conflicts of interest.

References

1 Diamond A: Executive functions. Annu Rev Clin Psychol 2014;64:135–168.
2 Georgieff MK: Nutrition and the developing brain: nutrient priorities and measurement. Am J Clin Nutr 2007;85:614S–620S.
3 Tanumihardjo SA, Russell RM, Stephensen CB, et al: Biomarkers of nutrition for development (BOND) – vitamin A review. J Nutr 2016;146: 1816S–1848S.
4 Stringham JM, Johnson EJ, Hammond BR: Lutein across the lifespan: from childhood cognitive performance to the aging eye and brain. Curr Dev Nutr 2019;3:nzz066.
5 Vishwanathan R, Kuchan MJ, Sen S, Johnson EJ: Lutein and preterm infants with decreased concentrations of brain carotenoids. J Pediatr Gastroenterol Nutr 2014;59:659–665.
6 Jeon S, Ranard KM, Neuringer M, et al: Lutein is differentially deposited across brain regions following formula or breast feeding of infant rhesus macaques. J Nutr 2018;148:31–39.
7 Bettler J, Zimmer JP, Neuringer M, Derusso PA: Serum lutein concentrations in healthy term infants fed human milk or infant formula with lutein. Eur J Nutr 2010;49:45–51.
8 Johnson EJ, Mcdonald K, Caldarella SM, et al: Cognitive findings of an exploratory trial of docosahexaenoic acid and lutein supplementation in older women. Nutr Neurosci 2008;11:75–83.
9 Renzi-Hammond L, Bovier E, Fletcher L, et al: Effects of a lutein and zeaxanthin intervention on cognitive function: a randomized, double-masked, placebo-controlled trial of younger healthy adults. Nutrients 2017;9:1246.
10 Lindbergh CA, Renzi-Hammond LM, Hammond BR, et al: Lutein and zeaxanthin influence brain function in older adults: a randomized controlled trial. J Int Neuropsychol Soc 2018;24:77–90.
11 McCorkle SM, Raine LB, Hammond BR, et al: Reliability of heterochromatic flicker photometry in measuring macular pigment optical density among preadolescent children. Foods 2015;4: 594–604.

12 Barnett SM, Khan NA, Walk AM, et al: Macular pigment optical density is positively associated with academic performance among preadolescent children. Nutr Neurosci 2018;21:632–640.
13 Walk AM, Khan NA, Barnett SM, et al: From neuro-pigments to neural efficiency: the relationship between retinal carotenoids and behavioral and neuroelectric indices of cognitive control in childhood. Int J Psychophysiol 2017;118:1–8.
14 Hassevoort KM, Khazoum SE, Walker JA, et al: Macular carotenoids, aerobic fitness, and central adiposity are associated differentially with hippocampal-dependent relational memory in preadolescent children. J Pediatr 2017;183:108–114.e1.
15 Bekdash RA: Choline, the brain and neurodegeneration: insights from epigenetics. Front Biosci (Landmark Ed) 2018;23:1113–1143.
16 Deoni SCL: Neuroimaging of the developing brain and impact of nutrition; in Colombo J, Koletzko B, Lampl M (eds): Recent Research in Nutrition and Growth. Nestlé Nutrition Institute Workshop Series. Basel, Karger, 2018, vol 89, pp 155–174.
17 Caudill MA, Strupp BJ, Muscalu L, et al: Maternal choline supplementation during the third trimester of pregnancy improves infant information processing speed: a randomized, double-blind, controlled feeding study. FASEB J 2018;32:2172–2180.
18 Edwards CG, Walk AM, Cannavale CN, et al: Dietary choline is related to neural efficiency during a selective attention task among middle-aged adults with overweight and obesity. Nutr Neurosci 2019, DOI: 10.1080/1028415X.2019.1623456.
19 Suh H, Kavouras SA: Water intake and hydration state in children. Eur J Nutr 2019;58:475–496.
20 Khan NA, Westfall DR, Jones AR, et al: A 4-d water intake intervention increases hydration and cognitive flexibility among preadolescent children. J Nutr 2019;149:2255–2264.
21 D'Anci KE, Constant F, Rosenberg IH: Hydration and cognitive function in children. Nutr Rev 2006;64:457–464.
22 Kempton MJ, Ettinger U, Foster R, et al: Dehydration affects brain structure and function in healthy adolescents. Hum Brain Mapp 2011;32:71–79.
23 Holscher HD: Dietary fiber and prebiotics and the gastrointestinal microbiota. Gut Microbes 2017;8:172–184.
24 Anderson JW, Baird P, Davis RH, et al: Health benefits of dietary fiber. Nutr Rev 2009;67:188–205.
25 Mohajeri MH, La Fata G, Steinert RE, Weber P: Relationship between the gut microbiome and brain function. Nutr Rev 2018;76:481–496.
26 Ticinesi A, Tana C, Nouvenne A, et al: Gut microbiota, cognitive frailty and dementia in older individuals: a systematic review. Clin Interv Aging 2018;13:1497–1511.
27 Rodríguez JM, Murphy K, Stanton C, et al: The composition of the gut microbiota throughout life, with an emphasis on early life. Microb Ecol Health Dis 2015;26:26050.
28 Vázquez E, Barranco A, Ramírez M, Gruart A, et al: Effects of a human milk oligosaccharide, 2′-fucosyllactose, on hippocampal long-term potentiation and learning capabilities in rodents. J Nutr Biochem 2015;26:455–465.
29 Khan NA, Raine LB, Drollette ES, et al: Dietary fiber is positively associated with cognitive control among prepubertal children. J Nutr 2015;145:143–149.
30 Desmedt O, Broers JV, Zamariola G, et al: Effects of prebiotics on affect and cognition in human intervention studies. Nutr Rev 2019;77:81–95.

Published online: November 9, 2020

Black MM, Singhal A, Hillman CH (eds): Building Future Health and Well-Being of Thriving Toddlers and Young Children. Nestlé Nutr Inst Workshop Ser. Basel, Karger, 2020, vol 95, pp 136–144 (DOI: 10.1159/000511511)

The Importance of Motor Skills for Development

Karen E. Adolph   Justine E. Hoch

Department of Psychology, New York University, New York, NY, USA

Abstract

Motor skills are important for development. Everything infants do involves motor skills – postural, locomotor, and manual actions; exploratory actions; social interactions; and actions with artifacts. Put another way, all behavior is motor behavior, and thus motor skill acquisition is synonymous with behavioral development. Age norms for basic motor skills provide useful diagnostics for "typical" development, but cultural differences in child-rearing practices influence skill onset ages. Whenever they emerge, motor skills lay the foundation for development by opening up new opportunities for learning. Postural control brings new parts of the environment into view and into reach; locomotion makes the larger world accessible; manual skills promote new forms of interactions with objects; and motor skills involving every part of the body enhance opportunities for social interaction. Thus, motor skills can instigate a cascade of developments in domains far afield from motor behavior – perception and cognition, language and communication, emotional expression and regulation, physical growth and health, and so on. Finally, motor skill acquisition makes behavior increasingly functional and flexible. Infants learn to tailor behavior to variations in their body and environment and to discover or construct new means to achieve their goals.

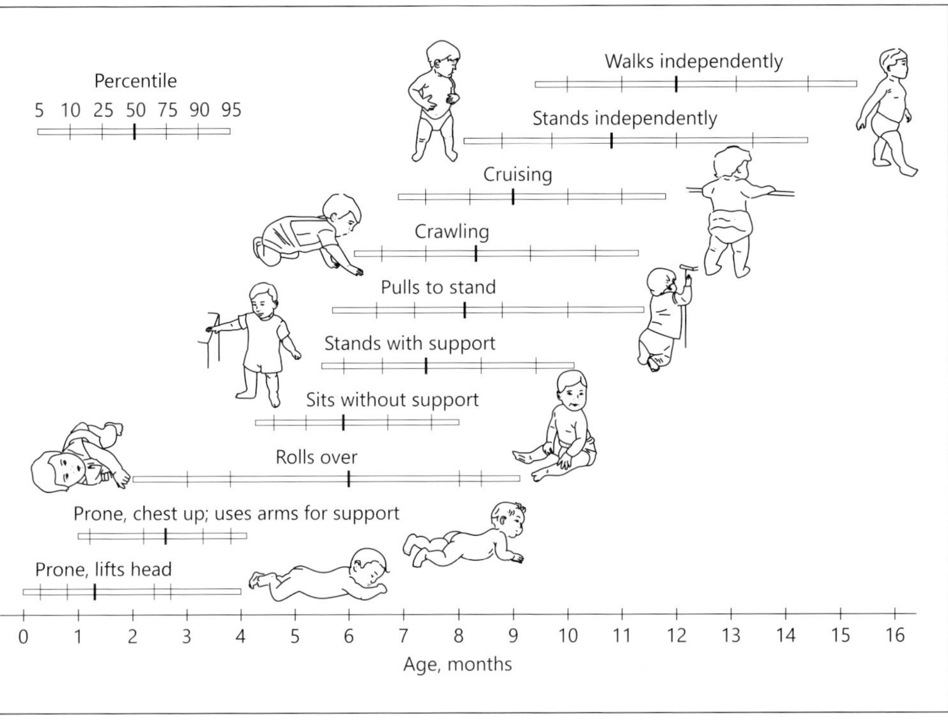

Fig. 1. Infant motor milestone chart. Line drawings and normative age bands show an age-related progression of motor skills. Age increases from left to right, and skills improve from bottom to top. The length of the horizontal bars represents the 5th to 95th percentiles; ticks denote the 10th, 25th, 50th, 75th, and 90th percentiles. Normative data for lifting the head while prone, propping the chest up while prone, rolling, and pulling to stand are from the Alberta Infant Motor Scale (AIMS). Data for sitting without support, crawling on hands and knees, cruising upright along furniture, standing while holding furniture, standing independently, and walking independently are from the WHO standards.

Motor Skill Acquisition Is Behavioral Development

Motor skills are important because they constitute infants' behaviors. People typically think of motor development as the items on a standard milestone chart: the parade of basic postural and locomotor skills from rolling and sitting to crawling, standing, and walking (Fig. 1). But milestone charts do not represent the scope of motor development. Infants' motor skills include every part of the body, from the eyes and other parts of the face down to the toes [for reviews, see 1–3]. Looking, smiling, suckling, eating, and using the mouth to "blow raspberries" and speak are all motor skills. Ditto for manual actions such as reaching, grasping, and exploring objects with hands and fingers, and likewise for actions with artifacts such as scribbling with a crayon, using a spoon, wielding a hammer, and pressing the buttons on a toy. Social and communicative actions (e.g., hugging a caregiver, petting a dog, pointing and nodding, or pretending to drink from a cup) also involve motor skills. Infant locomotion includes a mind-boggling array of behaviors – pivoting in circles, belly crawling, inchworming, bum shuffling, knee walking, log rolling, pulling to stand, cruising, sliding, backing, and climbing. Similarly, infants' postures (e.g., side-lying, mermaid posture, W-sit, ring-sit, long-sit, and short-sit positions) are so diverse that many postures commonly displayed by infants do not even have names.

In short, all behavior is motor behavior. Thus, to the extent that behavior is important, motor skills are important. Moreover, behavior develops. So, motor development is really behavioral development. From day to day, new skills enter and exit infants' repertoires, and frequently used skills continually improve [for reviews, see 1–3]. As illustrated in Figure 1, newborns are stuck with their head in the mattress; 18 months later, toddlers are racing across the living room floor. Newborns track a proffered block with their eyes, 4-month-old infants swat at it, 8-month-old infants grasp and explore it, and 18-month-old toddlers build block towers [4]. Banging the high chair tray transforms into hammering a peg [5]. Coos and babbles become fully articulated speech. The coordination between breathing and sucking to nurse is replaced with new patterns of coordination to chew and swallow solid foods [6]. Overall, motor skill acquisition reflects dramatic improvements in coordination, strength, balance control, and – given the diversity of infants' solutions – a great deal of ingenuity.

Motor Skills Reveal "Typical" Development

Motor skills are important because they provide a window into development. Generally, motor development is age related, as represented by the progression of skills in Figure 1. Age norms for skill onset provide a useful diagnostic tool because motor behavior is directly observable, skills are salient to caregivers and clinicians, and anomalies are correlated with many types of developmental disabilities. Indeed, most pediatricians' offices and parenting books contain a milestone chart or table of age norms, and when infants' onset ages fall beyond the normative range, clinicians and caregivers have cause for concern. The World Health Organization (WHO) even published "standards" (prescriptive age bands rather than descriptive norms) for infants' postural and locomotor milestones [7].

However, age norms must be interpreted with caution. Age and motor experience are highly correlated (older infants are also more experienced). When age and experience are unconfounded, experience trumps age as the key predictor

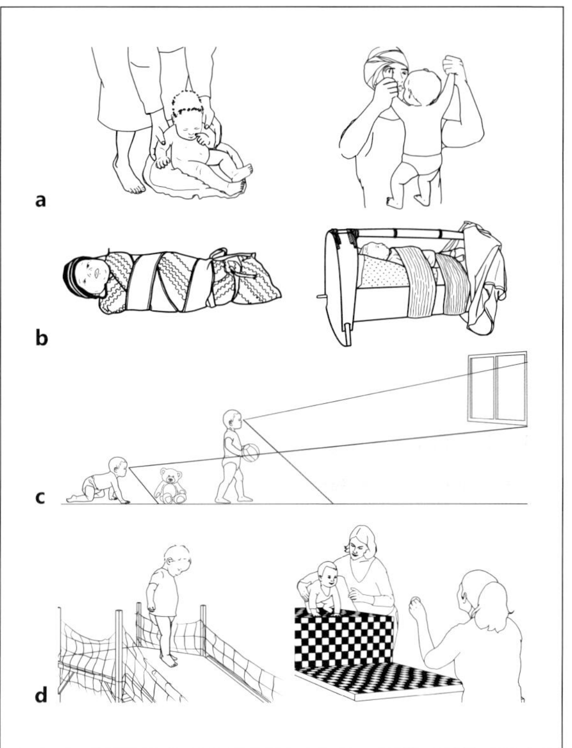

Fig. 2. a Examples of child-rearing practices that accelerate motor development. Left panel: Caregiver encouraging infant sitting. Right panel: Caregiver encouraging infant upright stepping. **b** Examples of child-rearing practices that delay motor development. Left panel: Tightly swaddled Quechua infant from Peru. Right panel: Infant from Tajikistan bound in a gahvora cradle. **c** Schematic drawing showing the enlargement in the average field of view for walking compared with crawling infants, and a greater propensity to carry toys. **d** Infants encountering obstacles. Left panel: Walking infant at the top of an adjustable slope. Right panel: Crawling infant at the precipice of an adjustable drop-off.

of skill emergence and improvement [for reviews, see 1–3]. The implications are twofold. First, motor skill acquisition is not a direct readout of neuromuscular maturation. Atypical development (earlier or later skill onset ages) reflects a history of motor experiences interacting with physiology. Second, because cultural differences in child-rearing practices affect infants' motor experiences, age norms should reflect worldwide diversity in child-rearing practices. But they do not. In Western and industrialized cultures, for example, caregivers handle newborns gently and support their head and trunk against gravity; caregivers allow infants freedom of movement through much of the 24-h day; and they expect infants' motor skills to develop naturally without special training. But such child-rearing practices are not universal.

In cultures that consider motor development as the result of exercise, caregivers deliberately train skills such as sitting and walking (Fig. 2a). Accordingly, infants achieve those milestones at earlier ages than would be expected based on western norms and the WHO standards [for reviews, see 1, 2, 8, 9]. Similarly, infants acquire postural and locomotor skills at earlier ages in cultures where caregivers use rough handling (lift babies by an arm or suspend infants by their ankles, for example), require infants to withstand gravity (e.g., hold infants without supporting their head), and expose infants to high-amplitude vestibular stimulation (e.g., carry them in slings while engaging in vigorous activities). Moreover, in experiments with random assignment to experimental and control groups, a few minutes of daily practice with upright stepping results in earlier onset of independent walking [10], and a few minutes of daily postural training leads to accelerated postural, manual, and locomotor skills [11].

Whereas most western caregivers assume that freedom to move is important for motor development, caregivers in some cultures do not [for reviews, see 1, 2, 8]. In rural China, caregivers bury supine infants up to their chests in sandbags [12], and in central Asia, caregivers bind infants neck to toe in a gahvora cradle for large parts of the 24-h day (Fig. 2b) [13]. Such constraint – even without social deprivation – delays postural and locomotor skills relative to western norms and the WHO standards. Even within the same culture, historical changes in child-rearing affect motor development. In western cultures, for example, the "Back to Sleep" campaign to put infants to sleep on their backs instead of their stomachs caused widespread delays in the emergence of rolling and crawling [14]. Merely wearing a diaper impedes walking compared with going naked, and old-fashioned cloth diapers present greater impediments than modern disposables [15].

Thus, attributions of "acceleration" or "delay" make sense only if the normative age bands include infants who experienced the same child-rearing practices. The first age norms were constructed from homogeneous groups of US infants. Although more racially and ethnically diverse, subsequent age norms and screening tests perpetuate the bias toward western, educated, middle-income populations [4]. The WHO standards [7] are based on data from 5 geographically, racially, and economically diverse countries (USA, Norway, India, Ghana, and Oman), but none have cultures that exercise or restrict infants' movements.

New Motor Skills Instigate Cascades of Development

As Piaget [16], Gibson [17], and others pointed out, motor skills are important because they lay the foundation for psychological development. The developmental story does not end with the ability to sit, walk, reach, and so on. New motor skills are only the beginning. Each motor achievement unlocks new parts of the environment for exploration and alters infants' interactions with objects, people, and places. New opportunities for learning, in turn, cascade into developments far afield from motor behavior [for reviews, see 1, 2, 8, 17, 18].

Advances in postural control literally broaden infants' world view. Before infants can lift their heads, their visual field is limited to what is already in sight [19]. Head control allows infants to decide for themselves what merits visual exploration. Sitting postural control expands infants' view to include the whole room and the people and objects in it [20]. The ability to crawl allows infants to see what is around the corner and in the next room [17]. The transition from crawling to walking provides even greater visual access to the environment (Fig. 2c). While crawling, infants mostly see the ground in front of their hands; while walking, they can spot far-off objects and places to explore [20].

The benefits of upright posture and walking do not end with improved visual access [for reviews, see 1, 2, 8]. Compared with crawling, walking infants spend more time in motion, travel farther distances, visit more places, access more distant objects, carry objects to new locations, and venture farther away from caregivers. Walkers are also more likely to carry objects to share with their caregivers, to initiate more joint engagement with caregivers, and to pay more attention to caregivers' gaze and points. Caregivers, in turn, are more likely to respond with language about what infants can do with the objects. Likely due to changes in language input, walking experience predicts infants' receptive and productive language, controlling for infants' age [21]. In addition, the onset of walking instigates surges in infant autonomy, self-efficacy, and control. Such links between locomotion and psychological development prompted a "mobility revolution" aimed at providing "ride-on cars" to children with disabilities to enable independent mobility [22].

Postural control also jump-starts a cascade of developments for manual actions [for reviews, see 1, 2]. Sitting postural control facilitates reaching, grasping, and visual-manual-oral object exploration. Object exploration, in turn, leads to new object knowledge. For example, infants with more sitting experience spontaneously produce more exploratory behaviors that reveal the three-dimensional form of objects. These exploration skills predict longer looking at displays that reveal unexpectedly hollow three-dimensional shapes [23]. Object exploration skills also facilitate cross-modal perception of object properties [24], discrimination of object boundaries [25], and mental rotation of objects [26]. Moreover, the ability to grasp objects (developed over time or experimentally boosted) helps infants understand the intent of others' manual actions [27].

Motor skill acquisition may also affect infants' body growth and health. Babies who move more have less belly fat [28]. But movement may also come at a cost. Crawling and walking momentarily churn up dust and debris, and some particles are detrimental if inhaled. Because crawlers' heads are so close to the

10 Zelazo PR, Zelazo NA, Kolb S: "Walking" in the newborn. Science 1972;176:314–315.
11 Lobo MA, Galloway JC: Enhanced handling and positioning in early infancy advances development throughout the first year. Child Dev 2012; 83:1290–1302.
12 Mei J: The northern Chinese custom of rearing babies in sandbags: implications for motor and intellectual development; in van Rossum JHA, Laszlo JI (eds): Motor Development: Aspects of Normal and Delayed Development. Amsterdam, VU Uitgeverij, 1994, pp 41–48.
13 Karasik LB, Tamis-LeMonda CS, Ossmy O, et al: The ties that bind: cradling in Tajikistan. PLoS One 2018;13:e0204428.
14 Davis BE, Moon RY, Sachs HC, et al: Effects of sleep position on infant motor development. Pediatrics 1998;102:1135–1140.
15 Cole WG, Lingeman JM, Adolph KE: Go naked: diapers affect infant walking. Dev Sci 2012;15: 783–790.
16 Piaget J: The Origins of Intelligence in Children. New York, International Universities Press, 1952.
17 Gibson EJ: Exploratory behavior in the development of perceiving, acting, and the acquiring of knowledge. Annu Rev Psychol 1988;39:1–41.
18 Campos JJ, Anderson DI, Barbu-Roth MA, et al: Travel broadens the mind. Infancy 2000;1:149–219.
19 Jayaraman S, Fusey CM, Smith LB: Why are faces denser in the visual experiences of younger than older infants? Dev Psychol 2017;53:38–49.
20 Kretch KS, Franchak JM, Adolph KE: Crawling and walking infants see the world differently. Child Dev 2014;85:1503–1518.
21 Walle EA, Campos JJ: Infant language development is related to the acquisition of walking. Dev Psychol 2014;50:336–348.
22 Logan SW, Hospodar CM, Feldner HA, et al: Modifed ride-on car use by young children with disabilities. Pediatr Phys Ther 2018;30:50–56.
23 Soska KC, Adolph KE, Johnson SP: Systems in development: motor skill acquisition facilitates three-dimensional object completion. Dev Psychol 2010;46:29–138.
24 Eppler MA: Development of manipulatory skills and the deployment of attention. Infant Behav Dev 1995;18:391–405.
25 Needham AW: Improvements in object exploration skills may facilitate the development of object segregation in early infancy. J Cogn Dev 2000;1:131–156.
26 Mohring W, Frick A: Touching up mental rotation: effects of manual experience on 6-month-old infants' mental object rotation. Child Dev 2013;84:1554–1565.
27 Sommerville JA, Woodward AL, Needham A: Action experience alters 3-month-old infants' perception of others' actions. Cognition 2005; 96:B1–B11.
28 Benjamin-Neelon SE, Bai J, Ostbye T, et al: Physical activity and adiposity in a racially diverse cohort of US infants. Obesity (Silver Spring) 2020; 28:631–637.
29 Wu T, Täubel M, Holopainen R, et al: Infant and adult inhalation exposure to resuspeded biological particulate matter. Environ Sci Technol 2018; 52:237–247.
30 Lampl M: Evidence of saltatory growth in infancy. Am J Hum Biol 1993;5:641–652.

Published online: November 9, 2020

Black MM, Singhal A, Hillman CH (eds): Building Future Health and Well-Being of Thriving Toddlers and Young Children. Nestlé Nutr Inst Workshop Ser. Basel, Karger, 2020, vol 95, pp 145–155 (DOI: 10.1159/000511512)

The Importance of Providing Opportunities for Health Behaviors during the School Day

Darla M. Castelli[a] Jeanne M. Barcelona[b] Brittany Crim[a] Sheri L. Burson[a]

[a]Department of Kinesiology and Health Education, The University of Texas at Austin, Austin, TX, USA; [b]College of Education, Wayne State University, Detroit, MI, USA

Abstract

Today, children are less active than previous generations leading to an increased prevalence of morbidity associated with physical inactivity. Globally, full-day preschool is rapidly becoming the norm. Thus, the amount of time that a child spends outside the home is an opportunity for schools and teachers to educate children about the importance of participating in physical activity and making healthy eating choices. One approach to comprehensively offer opportunities for physical activity and healthy eating is called *Whole School, Whole Community, Whole Child,* which intertwines academic success and promotion of healthy behaviors. Particularly for adolescent children, multicomponent approaches that include both school and family or community involvement have the most significant potential to make meaningful differences in the rate of physical activity participation. For young children, teacher training, resources, and equipment are needed to achieve equity across programs and schools, because these are predictors of physical activity participation. Further, school policies, administrative support, modeling by teachers, and the use of cues and incentives can have a positive effect. The purpose of this paper is to describe the benefits of contemporary, evidence-based models for providing opportunities for health behaviors in school from early childhood to adolescence.

Introduction

The World Health Organization (WHO) [1] asserts that unlike the previous generations, children today are mostly physically inactive. Alarmingly, young children exhibit low levels of physical activity that is far below the daily recommendation of 3 h of playtime for children under 5 years of age, and 60 min of moderate-to-vigorous physical activity for children aged 5–17 years. Such deficits occur because opportunities to move have been replaced with sedentary time [2]. Research suggests that Brazilian children ($n = 485$, mean age 10 years) spent approximately 56% of their waking hours in sedentary behavior (e.g., watching television) and only 2% of the time in vigorous physical activity [3]. The lack of time spent in moderate-to-vigorous physical activity was inversely related to body composition in boys, while girls were negatively impacted by a lack of time in vigorous physical activity and the amount of time spent in sedentary behavior. Since sedentary behaviors by themselves were not related to body composition, these findings suggest that even low-intensity physical activity may have some health benefits over sedentary time.

Physical activity only accounts for a portion of the modifiable behaviors involved in the prevention of excessive weight gain, and the risk for overweight or obesity, tooth decay, and juvenile diabetes during childhood, and cardiovascular disease and some cancers in later life. Establishing healthy eating patterns in young children (aged 3–4 years) is critical because micronutrients are required for brain development, and fewer than 1 in 10 adolescents eat the recommended amount of fruit and vegetables each day [4]. Unhealthy eating is further compounded by the consumption of sugar-sweetened beverages [5] and the fact that childhood obesity rates among minority groups are disproportionately higher than among non-Hispanic white children [6]. Given the prevalence of physical inactivity and unhealthy eating, the purpose of this paper is to describe the benefits of contemporary, evidenced-based models providing opportunities for health behaviors in school from early childhood to adolescence.

Key Findings among the Research

Globally, full-day preschool is rapidly becoming the norm, meaning 3- and 4-year-old children are joining children aged 5–18 years, who already spend 6 h a day in schools. The amount of time a child spends outside of the home is an opportunity for schools and teachers to educate children about the importance of participating in physical activity and making healthy eating choices; however, with the school curriculum already filled with academic requirements, little time is reserved for addressing such content and providing opportunities to participate.

Physical Activity in All Schools

Despite the known benefits of physical activity participation, across the world, physical inactivity is on the rise as technology has infiltrated daily tasks that require thus less energy expenditure than in previous generations who were needed to engage in manual labor for survival. The daily efficiency of transportation, employment, and education has been maximized through screen time and other conveniences. The current context may be placing children in a position where they are trading their active play and physical activity for time watching television or using a tablet, phone, or computer [7]. This is problematic, as screen time has been found to diminish the healthy development of the whole child, whereas physical activity has been found to promote it.

Physical activity in early childhood is often facilitated through structured and unstructured play [8]. Structured or guided play, known as play with a purpose [9], provides specific and planned activities that are tied to a given learning outcome. Unstructured play, also known as free play, provides the young child with opportunities to interact and explore their environment in a productive way that also engages social and emotional elements [10]. Physical activity guidelines indicate that young children should be engaging in ongoing physical activity throughout the day that includes both structured and unstructured play [2].

Structured play and movement opportunities in early childhood have been associated with cognitive and learning benefits. Research indicates that inhibition, or the ability to filter out classroom distractions to complete the task at hand, is significantly and positively influenced by physical activity regardless of intensity, suggesting that movement by itself enhances the young child's neural processing efficiency [11]. Further, physical activity that enhances gross motor coordination has been found to positively influence working memory and attention [12]. Classroom-based physical activity in the preschool setting has also been found to improve self-regulation and, in doing so, has improved academic readiness, or the young child's preparedness to take in new information [8, 13]. Among children in elementary school, single sessions of physical activity have been associated with increased cognitive performance [14], and regular participation has led to increased physical fitness [15], working memory [16], and inhibitory control [17]. Behaviorally, research supports the notion that the more movement a young child is provided, the more self-regulated [18] and attentive [19] they will be.

School Nutrition and Healthy Eating

While we know that physical activity participation is on the decline, other factors like unhealthy eating and low socioeconomic status also influence health [20]. Nutrient-dense, well-balanced meals are essential for proper growth, immunity, physical and cognitive development, health, and well-being. Eating patterns as a whole, i.e., the combinations of food and drinks that children consume, can impact body weight and the attainment of essential nutrients. Although the consumption of healthy eating, like fruits and vegetables, has long been a societal concern, changes in how foods are constructed, preserved, and prepared, like adding sugar to fruit drinks, have increased the risk for obesity. Although the WHO recommends that grown children limit intake of added sugars to 6 teaspoons per day or 5% of the total energy expenditure, consumption is influenced by the child's age and level of physical activity participation [21]. For example, in children 3 years of age, this would translate to less than 3 teaspoons. Globally, children and adolescents have consistently consumed more than 10% of their total calories from added sugars over the past 20 years. Also, research shows that children who consume the highest percentages of total calories from added sugars tend to consume the lowest amounts of nutrient-dense foods such as fruits and vegetables. All food and beverage choices matter as the appropriate caloric levels help to achieve healthy body weight, meet the nutrient needs of growing bodies, and reduce the risk of chronic diseases.

School-based interventions targeting healthy eating are most effective when paired with physical activity outcomes, when they provide accessibility to healthy food options, and when they restrict access to unhealthy food options [22]. Approaches that are customizable and focus on both the micro- (i.e., child) and macrosystems (i.e., school policies) [23] have the highest potential for impact; however, sometimes unintended consequences lead to new inequalities linked to socioeconomics.

A clustering of factors increases the health risk. Specifically, television watching for more than 1 h per day was associated with the consumption of fast foods, sweets, chips, and pizza, and reduced consumption of fruits and vegetables [24]. Moreover, this phenomenon was most prevalent among low socioeconomic families. To further our understanding, there needs to be increased scientific rigor among studies examining this phenomenon, e.g., in vulnerable minority populations.

Discussion

The intersectionality of socioecological systems identifies areas of overlap where a policy, e.g., to ban fried foods from school, could have both upstream and downstream effects. If french fries were replaced with fresh fruit, and recess was

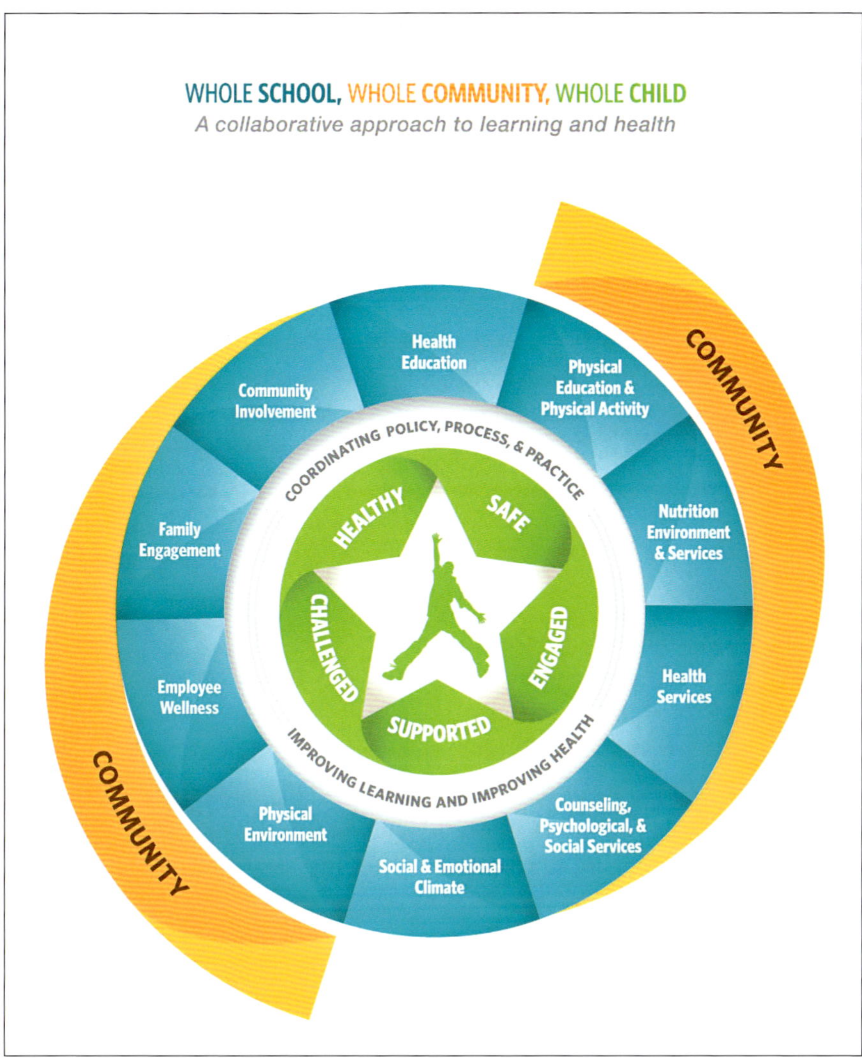

Fig. 1. The Whole School, Whole Community, Whole Child collaborative approach to learning and health [26].

offered before eating lunch, a child would have opportunities to learn how to make healthy choices. Further, by applying these strategies during early childhood education, benefits could be even greater as attending preschool is a significant predictor of physical activity [25]. Administrators, teachers, and families profit from the implementation of comprehensive health models such as the *Whole School, Whole Community, Whole Child* (WSCC) (Fig. 1) [26].

Whole School, Whole Community, Whole Child

"Health and education affect individuals, society, and the economy and, as such, must work together whenever possible. Schools are a perfect setting for collaboration" [26]. The WSCC intertwines academic success and prevalence of healthy behaviors, such as being regularly physically active and eating healthy. Models like WSCC identify points of intervention, provide justification for professional development for teachers and provision of resources, and help to develop strategies for overcoming barriers. In early childhood, the dosage and quality of the physical activity are dependent on the site. Several studies have investigated barriers to physical activity in child care settings citing issues ranging from lack of staff support and training to lack of space and resources [25]. In elementary and secondary schools, physical activity at school and healthy eating programs are often plagued by a lack of administrator support, school policies, teacher professional development, and few adults modeling healthy behaviors [27].

Student Access to Healthy Foods and Beverages at School

As part of the WSCC, the *Foods and Beverages in Schools Campaign* (Fig. 2) encourages teachers to provide healthy snacks at school, model healthy behaviors, and take advantage of healthy eating teaching opportunities [28]. The goals of this program include providing access to clean drinking water at no cost, providing 2 healthy school meals per day, integrating nutrition education into the school curriculum, and limiting access to unhealthy foods and beverages before, during, and after school.

Particularly for children and adolescents, multicomponent approaches that include both school and family or community involvement have the most significant potential to make meaningful differences in the rate of physical activity participation [3]. In early childhood, training teachers is a priority so that they can work toward acceptance of physical activity as a normative practice. When there was portable physical activity equipment, low use of technology, and large playground/activity spaces, children were less sedentary and spent more time in moderate-to-vigorous physical activity. These findings suggest that intentional modifications of the child care environment can promote increased physical activity. Specifically, teachers need to learn how to offer physical activity opportunities across the day. In elementary and secondary education, where children and adolescents have more agency, we might be guided by the Self-Determination Theory (SDT) to develop educational materials to support opportunities to be physically active and consume healthy snacks and meals.

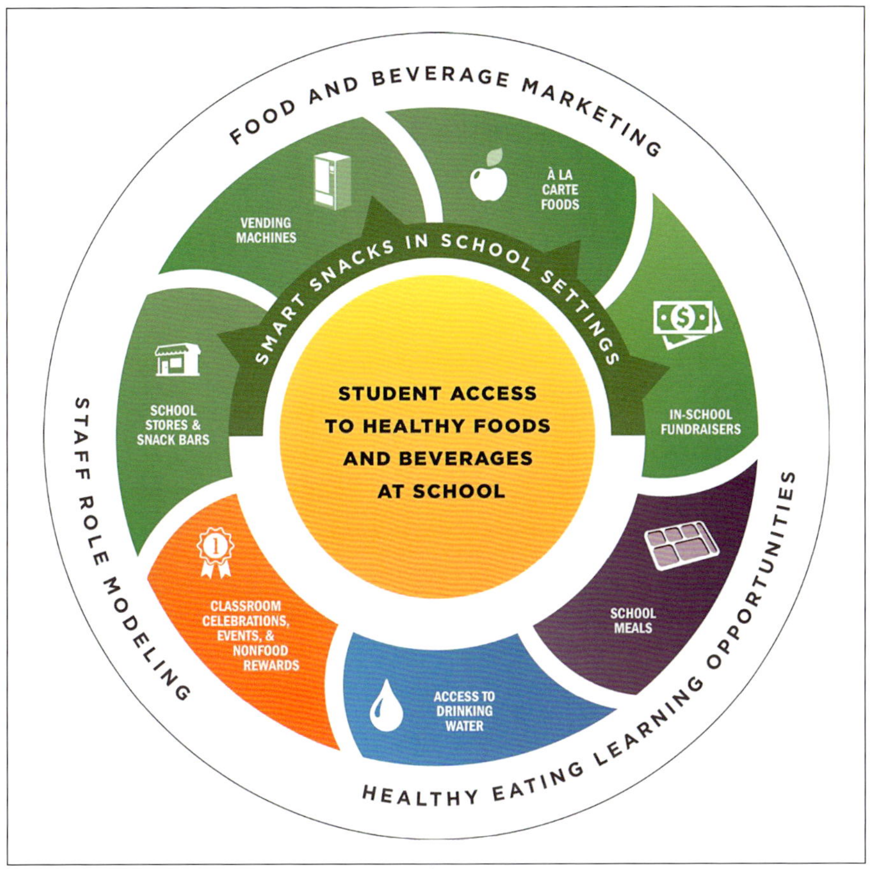

Fig. 2. Student access to healthy foods and beverages at school [26].

Self-Determination Theory

From a social cognitive perspective, SDT is commonly used to explain engagement and disengagement behaviors as intrinsic and extrinsic constructs of motivation [29]. Intrinsically motivated children play and move for enjoyment and satisfaction. Realistically, though, children sometimes need to be incentivized by offering them items of interest, such as rewards, to extrinsically motivate children to participate. SDT is grounded in 3 essential human psychological needs for competence, autonomy, and relatedness. These needs provide a fundamental source of mental energy for social behaviors manifested through human interactions in environments like classrooms, gymnasiums, and playgrounds [30]. *Competence* is the perception that one can complete a given task. Feelings of competence reflect satisfaction that often results from one's ability to produce the desired outcome and to demonstrate mastery. While *autonomy* is defined as the degree to which indi-

Table 1. Evidence-based practices for physical activity and nutrition at school

Who is responsible?	What needs to occur?	How do children benefit?
Administrators as policy makers	Invest in improving student health	Healthy children are more ready to learn
Administrators as financial stewards	Provide regular opportunities for professional development	Healthy and well-trained teachers are more ready to help children learn
Teachers as health promoters	Make health-first decisions Offer nourishing snacks like air-popped popcorn, fresh fruits, yogurt, and whole-grain foods	Child-centered approaches meeting the child where they are at
Teachers as continual learners	Participate in professional development focused on child health, how to offer physical activity safely, and increase student knowledge about healthy eating	Children experience innovative teaching and comprehensive models
Teachers as health champions	Support and encourage a sustained culture of health Provide opportunities to try new foods Limit added sugar as rewards	Children will follow their adult and peer models Child have a chance to practice healthy decision-making
Teachers as practitioners	Intentional teaching practices that embed routine physical activity and drinking water across the school day	Habitual physical activity and healthy eating will reduce health risk: both improve immediate and long-term cognitive performance
Teachers as organizers	Use learning activities to make healthy decisions	Opportunities to be active and make healthy choices before, during, and after school can create habits
Parents as providers	Parental engagement that reinforces healthy eating and physical activity at home: reduce fast-food consumption; be active as a family; and model healthy eating behaviors	Community connections can support children to make healthy choices
Administrators, teachers, and parents	Engaging youth in health leadership opportunities that provide them with a say and a voice	Listen to the voices of children: "Mom, can you please bring home some fruit?" "Ms. Arrendo, can we go outside today?" Mr. Oliverio, can we get a salad bar as part of our school lunch?"

viduals perceive themselves as the origin or source responsible for the initiation of the behavior, *relatedness* is the extent to which individuals feel connected to others through activities and their sense of belonging both to their community and other individuals. The application of SDT to school-based interventions allows us to differentiate between goals and self-regulatory processes like health behaviors. The underlying assumptions of the SDT are (a) a school/parent-initiated environment can influence the formation of motivational regulations and (b) motivational regulations have cognitive, affective, and behavioral outcomes. These assumptions are behaviorally carried out as self-regulation.

Implications

Administrators, teachers, parents, and children have roles in promoting and supporting regular participation in physical activity and healthy eating (Table 1). Administrators need to invest in children's health and the training of teachers to provide opportunities for physical activity before, during, and after school, as healthier children are more ready to learn. By financing professional development for teachers and securing the resources necessary for implementing the WSCC framework, there is a potential for children to learn how to make healthy choices. Administrators can establish an expectation for building a health-enhancing school climate.

From this health-first perspective, teachers, once trained, are positioned to be both practitioners and health promoters [31]. Pedagogical steps for increasing the potential for healthy decision-making, based on the SDT, would suggest the following evidenced-based practices. First, teachers could provide educational experiences wherein children learn about the importance of their health and how to make healthy choices. Teachers need to differentiate activities for varying abilities so that everyone can be optimally challenged at his or her own level and achieve success. Next, teachers need to praise students for the effort they put into the learning processes rather than just for the outcomes. In other words, teachers should create a mastery climate focused more on the acquisition of decision-making skills and self-regulation. Since health behaviors are organic, continual, positive feedback can help children to improve their competence.

Table 1 summarizes these strategies and outlays the benefits for children and adolescents. Physical education can be an ideal place for increasing relatedness, as there is often more time compared to classroom experiences dedicated to practice and gameplay. Cooperative and team activities are opportunities for relatedness to emerge. Having affiliation and being connected to school or a class like physical education can be a powerful predictor of student engagement.

A relatively novel approach is to include the students' voices and give them a say in the development of authentic learning experiences. Student choice increases perceived control over their own health behaviors. During physical education, there was a positive association between perceived competence and self-regulation [30]. If students are capable of applying self-regulation strategies, in theory, they should be able to develop and maintain the motivation to carry out healthful living. When teachers utilize these strategies, there are typically positive learning outcomes for children and adolescents.

Conflict of Interest Statement

The authors declare no known conflicts of interest.

References

1 World Health Organization: World Health Statistics 2019: Monitoring Health for the SDGs, sustainable development goals. Geneva, WHO, 2019.

2 Hnatiuk JA, Salmon J, Hinkley T, et al: A review of preschool children's physical activity and sedentary time using objective measures. Am J Prev Med 2014;47:487–497.

3 de Moraes Ferrari GL, Oliveira LC, Araujo TL, et al: Moderate-to-vigorous physical activity and sedentary behavior: independent associations with body composition variables in Brazilian children. Pediatr Exerc Sci 2015;27:380–389.

4 Gidding SS, Dennison BA, Birch LL, et al; American Heart Association: Dietary recommendations for children and adolescents: a guide for practitioners. Pediatrics 2006;117:544–559.

5 Keller A, Bucher Della Torre S: Sugar-sweetened beverages and obesity among children and adolescents: a review of systematic literature reviews. Childhood Obes 2015;11:338–346.

6 Hales CM, Carroll MD, Fryar CD, et al: Prevalence of obesity among adults and youth: United States, 2015–2016. NCHS Data Brief 2017;288: 1–8.

7 Duch H, Fisher EM, Ensari I, Harrington A: Screen time use in children under 3 years old: a systematic review of correlates. Int J Behav Nutr Phys Act 2013;10:102.

8 Becker DR, McClelland MM, Loprinzi P, Trost SG: Physical activity, self-regulation, and early academic achievement in preschool children. Early Educ Dev 2014;25:56–70.

9 Danniels E, Pyle A: Defining play-based learning; in Tremblay RE, Boivin M, Peters RDeV, (eds), Pyle A (topic ed): Encyclopedia on Early Childhood Development [online]. 2018. http://www.child-encyclopedia.com/play-based-learning/according-experts/defining-play-based-learning.

10 Burdette HL, Whitaker RC: A national study of neighborhood safety, outdoor play, television viewing, and obesity in preschool children. Pediatrics 2005;116:657–662.

11 Pesce C, Masci I, Marchetti R, et al: Deliberate play and preparation jointly benefit motor and cognitive development: mediated and moderated effects. Front Psychol 2019;7:349.

12 Piek JP, Dawson L, Smith LM, Gasson N: The role of early fine and gross motor development on later motor and cognitive ability. Hum Mov Sci 2008;27:668–681.

13 Toumpaniari K, Loyens S, Mavilidi MF, Paas F: Preschool children's foreign language vocabulary learning by embodying words through physical activity and gesturing. Educ Psychol Rev 2015;27: 445–456.

14 Hillman CH, Pontifex MB, Raine L, et al: The effect of acute treadmill walking on cognitive control and academic achievement in preadolescent children. Neuroscience 2009;159:1044–1054.

15 Castelli DM, Hillman CH, Hirsch J, et al: FIT kids: time in target heart zone and cognitive performance. Prev Med 2011;52 suppl 1: S55–S59.

16 Kamijo K, Pontifex M, O'Leary KC, et al: The effects of an afterschool physical activity program on working memory in preadolescent children. Dev Sci 2011;14:1046–1058.

17 Drollette ES, Pontifex MB, Raine LB, et al: Effects of the FITKids physical activity randomized controlled trial on conflict monitoring in youth. Psychophysiology 2018;55:10.1111/psyp.13017.
18 Robinson LE, Palmer KK, Bub KL: Effect of the children's health activity motor program on motor skills and self-regulation in head start preschoolers: an efficacy trial. Front Public Health 2016;4:173.
19 Holmes RM, Pellegrini AD, Schmidt SL: The effects of different recess timing regimens on preschoolers' classroom attention. Early Child Dev Care 2006;176:735–743.
20 Müller MJ, Koertzinger I, Mast M, et al: Physical activity and diet in 5 to 7 years old children. Public Health Nutr 1999;2(suppl 3a):443–444.
21 World Health Organization: Guideline: Sugars Intake for Adults and Children. Geneva, WHO, 2015.
22 De Bourdeaudhuij I, van Cauwenberghe E, Spittaels H, et al: School-based interventions promoting both physical activity and healthy eating in Europe: a systematic review within the HOPE project. Obes Rev 2011;12:205–216.
23 McGill R, Anwar E, Orton L, et al: Are interventions to promote healthy eating equally effective for all? Systematic review of socioeconomic inequalities in impact. BMC Public Health 2015;15;457.
24 Finn K, Johannsen N, Specker B: Factors associated with physical activity in preschool children. J Pediatr 2020;140:81–85.
25 Tandon PS, Garrison MM, Christakis DA: Physical activity and beverages in home- and center-based child care programs. J Nutr Educ Behav 2012;44:355–359.
26 ASCD and Centers for Disease Control and Prevention [CDC]: Whole School, Whole Community, Whole Child: A Collaborative Approach to Learning and Health. Alexandria/Atlanta, ACS/CDC, 2014. http://www.ascd.org/ASCD/pdf/siteASCD/publications/wholechild/wscc-a-collaborative-approach.pdf.
27 Wechsler H, Devereaux RS, Davis M, Collins J: Using the school environment to promote physical activity and healthy eating. Prev Med 2000;31:S121–S137.
28 Centers for Disease Control and Prevention [CDC]: School Nutrition. Atlanta, CDC, 2019. https://www.cdc.gov/healthyschools/nutrition/schoolnutrition.htm.
29 Ryan RM, Deci EL: Intrinsic and extrinsic motivations: classic definitions and new directions. Contemp Educ Psychol 2000;25:54–67.
30 Sun H: Motivation as a learning strategy; in Ennis CD (ed): Routledge Handbook of Physical Education Pedagogies. New York, Routledge, 2017.
31 Castelli DM, Centeio EE, Nicksic HM: Preparing educators to promote and provide physical activity in schools. Am J Lifestyle Med 2013;7:324–332.

Published online: November 6, 2020

Black MM, Singhal A, Hillman CH (eds): Building Future Health and Well-Being of Thriving Toddlers and Young Children. Nestlé Nutr Inst Workshop Ser. Basel, Karger, 2020, vol 95, pp 156–159 (DOI: 10.1159/000511520)

Summary on Health Behaviors and the Developing Brain

The 4 articles provided in this last session entitled "Health Behaviors and the Developing Brain" stem from the 95th Nestlé Nutrition Institute Workshop, which took place virtually due to the Covid-19 pandemic in September 2020. The authors were brought together as a function of their common research focus on the influence of various health factors and lifestyle behaviors on the developing brain. As can be seen from the collection of articles, each is focused on a set of distinct, yet related, health factors that affect brain development (i.e., brain structure or function), as observed via alterations in cognitive or behavioral outcomes. To that end, the 4 articles represent a cohesive collection that provides a window into lifestyle factors that may shape health and wellness during childhood and across the lifespan.

Prior to summarizing each of the articles, it is worth revisiting the concept of critical periods of development, which is inherent in each of the health factors discussed and can be used as a means to frame a common theme across articles. A critical period refers to a specific time during development when the brain is especially plastic and susceptible to environmental exposures (i.e., amenable to molding or remodification). Although considerably more is known about how critical periods of development relate to other behaviors (e.g., language acquisition or visually guided actions), little evidence for the specific effects of health and lifestyle factors during critical periods of development has been demonstrated in the human literature. Despite the concept of critical periods of development being a guiding principle in our understanding of health and lifestyle factors on brain development, our understanding is also, to date, largely theoretical. Regardless, the implications of specific developmental periods are evident for the health and effective function of individuals as they progress through the lifespan.

Accordingly, the article by Adolph and Hoch provides insight into motor skill acquisition and brain development during infancy and early childhood. As the authors indicate, everything that infants do involves motor skills – postural, locomotor, and manual actions, as well as exploratory actions, social interactions, and interactions with objects and places in the environment. All behavior involves motor action, so motor skill acquisition is essential for healthy functioning. Moreover, because motor behavior both relies on and facilitates typical brain development, motor skills can serve as a marker of health or dysfunction. Although many people assume that basic motor skills (e.g., sitting and walking) are the outcome of neuromuscular maturation, environmental influences play a critical role in the development of motor behavior. Motor skills are shaped by culture. Thus, within a culture (i.e., a particular environment), age norms for motor skill acquisition are diagnostic of typical development, but across cultures, onset ages are less diagnostic due to differences in child-rearing practices. For example, cultural differences in onset ages of sitting and walking reflect differences in how caregivers hold, handle, dress, carry, and exercise their infants, and how they structure infants' environments. Nonetheless, regardless of onset age, new motor behaviors create new opportunities for learning. For example, Adolph and Hoch eloquently state: "Postural control brings new parts of the environment into view and into reach; locomotion makes the larger world accessible; manual skills promote new forms of interactions with objects; and motor skills involving every part of the body enhance opportunities for social interaction. Thus, motor skills can instigate a cascade of developments in domains far afield from motor behavior – perception and cognition, language and communication, emotional expression and regulation, physical growth and health, and so on."

The development of motor skill acquisition provides a foundation for physically active behaviors across childhood and the lifespan. Hillman, McDonald, and Logan summarize the effects of physical activity and physical fitness on cognition and brain health across childhood and adolescence. At a time when the majority of children do not meet physical activity guidelines, it is imperative that the health implications of inactivity are understood to develop adequate interventions and best provide public health recommendations. However, our understanding of the benefits of physical activity for brain and cognition (including academic achievements) varies across childhood and adolescence. That is, most of our knowledge is based on research with preadolescent children (6–13 years of age), with considerably less known about preschool-age children (<6 years) and adolescents (14–18 years). Regardless, the findings indicate that physical activity is especially beneficial for executive functions – the set of cognitive processes involved in the selection, scheduling, and coordination of goal-directed thoughts and actions, including inhibition, working memory, and mental flexibility. Importantly, executive functions underlie aspects of academic achievement, including mathematics and language skills, which also benefit from physical activity. Furthermore, specific brain regions and neural networks that underpin executive processes show benefits in structure and function from physical activity or greater amounts of aerobic fitness. Thus, physical activity and higher aerobic fitness beneficially affect the neural and cognitive processes that support academic achievement in school-age children.

Relatedly, Willis and Khan review the literature on the relationship between nutrition and cognition in children. Nutrition plays a fundamental role in the development of brain structure and function and has the potential to affect cognition through the provision of essential nutrients for brain development, serving as precursors to neurotransmitters, amelioration of neuroinflammation, and as a source of energy, for example. Furthermore, decrements in essential nutrients negatively impact cognition and brain function. However, relatively little is known about the role of overall diet quality in promoting cognitive health among children in the absence of nutrient deficits. Interestingly, Willis and Khan provided evidence that greater adherence to the recommended US dietary guidelines and other composite indices is associated with superior executive function in school-age children. Further evidence indicates that a relationship between overall diet quality and cognition is evident in children by 4 years of age, suggesting the influence of proper nutrition on cognition in early childhood. Moreover, key nutrients such as water, choline, lutein, and dietary fiber known to characterize higher-quality diets proffer specific benefits to executive function and memory; however, future work in children is warranted using causal models such as randomized controlled trials. Nevertheless, emerging evidence suggests that key nutrients support executive function in children. Given that nutritional recommendations for childhood cognition are absent from the US dietary guidelines, such findings may inform public health models related to the provision of healthy meals during the school day.

With a more applied focus, Castelli, Barcelona, Crim, and Burson discuss the literature on the provision of health behaviors, including physical activity and nutritional opportunities, during the school day. Currently, children spend large parts of their weekdays in school, so the importance of administrators and educators in supporting and modeling health behaviors is increasingly important. To that end, Castelli et al. describe the *Whole School, Whole Community, Whole*

Child framework, which provides opportunities for meeting recommended daily goals for moderate-to-vigorous physical activity and incorporates a larger, multicomponent (i.e., school, family, and community) view of achieving health behaviors (i.e., physical activity and healthy eating) and having academic success. The overarching belief of the *Whole School, Whole Community, Whole Child* model is that healthier children are better learners, because of the cognitive benefits and improved brain health that stem from engagement and commitment to healthy lifestyle choices. As such, ample opportunity for engagement is necessary, such that both structured and unstructured play, movement, physical education, recess, sport, and the provision of appealing, nutritious foods should be integrated into children's daily lives. Such an approach offers opportunities to be physically active and learn about the importance of making healthy choices, reduces health risks, and improves readiness for learning.

In summary, health behaviors such as physical activity and nutritional intake are essential to optimal brain development. Such behaviors in early childhood impact health and effective function across development and into adulthood. The building blocks of motor skill acquisition and provision of key nutrients are fundamental to the development of physical activity behaviors and healthy eating during childhood and adolescence, which have demonstrated benefits for brain health, cognition, and academic achievements. Although more research is needed to understand when to intervene (i.e., critical periods of development) and what types of intervention may be most effective, a growing literature indicates that health behaviors benefit brain and cognition, as well as real-world outcomes, including academic achievements, across childhood and adolescence.

Charles H. Hillman

Subject Index